Mauricio de Maio & Berthold Rzany

**Botulinum Toxin in Aesthetic Medicine**

Mauricio de Maio & Berthold Rzany

# Botulinum Toxin
# in Aesthetic Medicine

With 151 Figures and 36 Tables

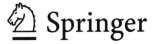 Springer

Editors

**B. Rzany**
Professor of Dermatology
Clinical Epidemiologist, Division of Evidence Based Medicine (dEBM)
Klinik für Dermatologie
CHARITÉ – UNIVERSITÄTSMEDIZIN BERLIN
Charitéplatz 1
10117 Berlin, Germany

**M. de Maio**
Plastic Surgeon
Faculty of Medicine of the University of São Paulo
Av. Ibirapuera, 2907 – cj. 1202
Moema – São Paulo – SP
CEP: 04029-200, Brazil

ISBN      978-3-540-34094-2    Springer Berlin Heidelberg New York

Library of Congress Control Number: 2006938423

Springer-Verlag is a part of Springer Science+Business Media
springer.com

© Springer-Verlag Berlin Heidelberg 2007

Editor: Marion Philipp, Heidelberg, Germany
Desk Editor: Ellen Blasig, Heidelberg, Germany
Cover design: Frido Steinen-Broo, eStudio Calamar, Spain
Typesetting and Production: LE-TEX Jelonek, Schmidt & Vöckler GbR, Leipzig, Germany

Printed on acid-free paper   24/3180/YL   5 4 3 2 1   SPIN 12190119

# Foreword

## Botulinumtoxin A in Aesthetic Medicine

Gary D. Monheit, M.D.

Probably the most important event in the evolution of minimally invasive cosmetic procedures is the development of botulinum toxin for cosmetic usage. From a single region and procedure for the treatment of the frown lines over a decade ago, the use of botulinum toxin has evolved into multiple areas, techniques, dosages and now new toxins in this ever expanding field. To capture it all in a comprehensive yet easily read and organized text, Drs de Maio and Rzany have put together this new volume in their approach to facial cosmetics.

This is a welcome addition to their first text on injectable fillers in Aesthetic Medicine. It is organized in a similar fashion, first giving an overview of the toxin discussing pharmacochemistry, sub-types and products, efficacy, dosage, effectiveness and finally safety. The clinical applications are divided into patient selection, basic requirements and injection techniques. The unique approach of correlating individual anatomic differences in patients as to dosage and injection points with muscle mass gives the clinician a new guide to successful treatment. The technique injection sections discuss all the treatable areas from upper face to lower face and neck, covering anatomy, treatment aims, patient selection, technique, complications and "tips and tricks".

In this text the clinician will find a wealth of information collected over years of experience by these two renowned aesthetic researchers and clinicians. I highly recommend this text for all aesthetic clinicians from the novice to those with years of experience as the learning curve is applicable for all.

Gary D. Monheit, MD
Clinical Associate Professor
Departments of Ophthalmology and Dermatology
University of Alabama at Birmingham
Dermatology Associates, Ash Place
Suite 202, 2100 16th Avenue South, Birmingham
AL, 35205, USA

# Foreword

Christopher Rowland Payne

No cosmetic item has had more impact than botulinum toxin. It is a worldwide phenomenon that has revolutionised cosmetic practice since its introduction 15 years ago. It is almost impossible to find any issue of a women's magazine from the last ten years which does not include a mention of botulinum toxin. This tsunami of interest amongst the public and amongst physicians has brought forth advances in the way in which botulinum toxin can be used to benefit the face cosmetically. At the crest of this wave of innovation are a number of notable doctors. Amongst this select group are Mauricio de Maio and Berthold Rzany. Their own original work on botulinum has achieved peer admiration around the world. They are known not only for the quality of their scientific papers but also for the clarity of their presentations at scientific and clinical meetings and they each have a huge personal following of loyal patients.

Accordingly, it is absolutely apposite that Mauricio de Maio and Berthold Rzany should be publishing this book now. It is their second book and will bring the practitioner reader right up to date. They discuss the movement away from "more is more" towards "individualisation and the microinjection technique". The text emphasises clinical method and clearly outlines "how to do it", making elegant use of half and half (before and after) facial photography of the highest standard. Photographs of this sort require enormous care and patience. Practitioners – and also potential patients – will greatly appreciate these illustrations.

Important discussion points are covered in a 'questions and answers' section, including the thorny question of the frequency with which injections need to be repeated. The text, which is fully referenced and, where possible evidence-based, also covers the more advanced and most recent uses of botulinum, including the botulinum face lift, the treatment of facial asymmetry and, of course, safety considerations, contraindications and so on.

This book fully deserves to become the *vade mecum* of aesthetic botulinum toxin.

Christopher Rowland Payne
Secretary-General (& Past President) of the European Society
of Cosmetic & Aesthetic Dermatology

London
January 2007

# Preface

Why another book on botulinum toxin in aesthetic medicine? There are a couple of reasons. First: the main reason is the tremendous progress that we are seeing in the use of this drug, which rapidly outstrips the present literature. Second: we still think there is a need for good books as there is still a lot of confusion and misconceptions around the different indications and the different drugs.

Unlike in the beginning, when botulinum toxin A was used along the principles of 'the same injection points and doses for everybody' and 'bigger doses for bigger effects' it is now used in a much more differentiated way. Based on the muscular patterns (kinetic, hyperkinetic and hypertonic), we have a much more individualized approach to the treatment of our patients. New indications in the middle and lower third of the face have been added to the well-known areas of the upper face. Multiple facial areas are now treated during one visit, with the aim of global facial rejuvenation with the ultimate aim of the botulinum toxin 'face lift'. Besides the classic intramuscular injection technique, microinjection techniques are increasingly used. Furthermore, the botulinum toxin world is not a two-product world any more. More and more botulinum toxin products are entering the field to fight for their share in the market.

Based on the views of a plastic surgeon and a dermatologist, this book aims to familiarize the novice as well as skilled user with these new concepts and new preparations to enable both to treat their patients in the best possible way.

This book complements our book on injectable fillers in aesthetic medicine. Like our first book, we have followed an honest 'how we do it' approach. As our aim is to improve our teachings we always appreciate direct feedback from our readers, and we encourage you to give us your comments and suggestions for improvement.

Berlin and Sao Paulo, August 2006

Mauricio de Maio    Berthold Rzany

# Acknowledgments

Neither our first, nor this, our second book, would have been possible without the work of many others. We would therefore like to take the opportunity to thank our patients who helped us get to where we are now, especially those who contributed their photographs to this book. At Springer, we would like to thank Mrs. Marion Philipp and Mrs. Ellen Blasig, and from the German team: Mr. Hendrik Zielke for his help with the content and format, especially for helping us build the chapters on the efficacy and safety of the different botulinum toxin preparations and his ability to cope with all the software, and Mr. Tobias Gottermeier for the excellent photographs and graphic work.

From the Brazilian team: Mrs. Emma Mattos for helping with the updated references of botulinum toxin treatments; Mrs. Liliann Amoroso for working on the photo library which was quite tiring and demanding; and especially the clinical assistants Mrs. Gisele Souza, Mrs. Liliane Carneiro, Mrs. Renata Sanches and Mr. Thais Sorcinelli who have a wonderfully careful way with my patients.

# Contents

# List of Contributors

**Berthold Rzany MD ScM**
Professor of Dermatology
Clincial Epidemiologist

**Hendrik Zielke MD**
Email: hendrik.zielke@charite.de
Division of Evidence Based Medicine (dEBM)
Klinik für Dermatologie
CHARITÉ – UNIVERSITÄTSMEDIZIN
BERLIN
CAMPUS CHARITÉ MITTE
Charitéplatz 1
D - 10117 Berlin
Germany

Phone: 0049 (0)30 - 450518 - 283
Fax: 0049 (0)30 - 450518 - 927
Email: berthold.rzany@charite.de
http://www.debm.de or www.rzany-berlin.de

**Mauricio de Maio MD, PhD, MSc**
Plastic Surgeon
Faculty of Medicine of the University of Sao
Paulo
Av. Ibirapuera, 2907 - cj. 1202
Moema - São Paulo - SP
CEP: 04029-200
Brazil

Phone/fax: 0055 11 55359286
Email: mauriciodemaio@uol.com.br

# List of Abbreviations

**BNT**    Botulinum toxin

**EADV**   European Academy of Dermatology and Venerology

**EBM**    Evidence Based Medicine

**MU**     Mouse units

# Chapter 1

# Overview of Botulinum Toxin

Berthold Rzany, Hendrik Zielke

1

## Contents

## 1.1 Introduction

Botulinum toxin (BNT) is a fascinating drug which specifically targets the release of acetylcholine. BNT is produced by the anaerobic bacterium *Clostridium botulinum*. In order to be used as a drug the toxin has to be isolated, purified and stabilized (Huang et al. 2000) (Table 1.1).

## 1.2 Different Subtypes of Botulinum Toxin

Seven distinct antigenic botulinum toxins (BNT-A, -B, -C, -D, -E, -F, and -G) produced by different strains of *Clostridium botulinum* have been described. The human nervous system is susceptible to five toxin serotypes (BNT-A, -B, -E, -F, -G) and unaffected by 2 (BNT-C, -D). Although all toxins have different molecular targets, their action leads to the blockade of the cholinergic nerves. However, only the A and B toxins are available as drugs. In aesthetic medicine, the BNT predominately used has been of type A so far, even though some trials have been published utilizing type B BNT (Baumann et al. 2003).

## 1.3 Mode of Action

BNT blocks the action of acetylcholine. Acetylcholine is a common neural transmitter and

**Table 1.1.** Pharmacological aspects of therapeutic botulinum toxin preparations (modified from Dressler 2006)

| | Botox/Vistabel | Dysport | Xeomin | Myobloc/NeuroBloc |
|---|---|---|---|---|
| Manufacturer | Allergan, Inc Irvine, CA, USA | Ipsen Ltd. Slough, Berks, UK | Merz Pharmaceuticals Frankfurt/M, Germany | Elan Plc. Dublin, Ireland |
| Pharmaceutical form | powder | powder | powder | solution for injection |
| Storage precautions | below 8°C | below 8°C | below 25°C | below 8°C |
| Shelf life | 24 months | 15 months | 36 months | 24 months |
| Botulinum-toxin-serotype | A | A | A | B |
| *Clostridium-botulinum-* strain | Hall A | Ipsen strain | Hall A | Bean B |
| SNARE-target of action | SNAP25 | SNAP25 | SNAP25 | VAMP |
| Purification | precipitation and chromatography | precipitation and chromatography | precipitation and chromatography | precipitation and chromatography |
| pH-value of the reconstituted preparation | 7.4 | 7.4 | 7.4 | 5.6 |
| Stabilization | vacuum drying | freeze drying (lyophilization) | vacuum drying | pH-reduction |
| Excipients | human serum albumin 500 µg/vial NaCl 900 µg/vial | human serum albumin 125 µg/vial lactose 2500 µg/vial | human serum albumin 1 mg/vial sucrose 5 mg/vial | human serum albumin 500 µg/ml NaCl 6 mg/ml |
| Biological activity | 100 MU-A/vial or 50 MU-A/vial | 500 MU-I/vial | 100 MU-M/vial | 5.0 kMU-E/ml as 2.5/5.0/10.0 kMU-E /vial |
| Biological activity in relation to Botox | 1 | 1/3 | 1 | 1/40 |
| Molecular weight of the BNT component | 900 kD | 900 kD | 150 kD | 600 kD |

**BNT botulinum-neurotoxin,** MU-A mouse-unit in the Allergan-mouse lethality assay, MU-E mouse-unit in the Elan-mouse lethality assay, MU-I mouse-unit in the Ipsen-mouse lethality assay, MU-M mouse-unit in the Merz-mouse lethality assay

stimulates striated as well as smooth muscles and the secretion of glands such as sweat glands.

After BNT has been ingested or injected, it diffuses into the human tissue until it selectively and irreversibly binds to the presynaptic terminal of the neuromuscular or neuroglandular junction, where it exerts its actions by cleaving specific membrane proteins responsible for acetylcholine excretion.

It is important to understand that the action of the BNT does not occur immediately. Usually the maximum effect can be seen after a couple of weeks. The first effects might be visible after 48 hours. Depending on the strength of the muscles treated and the dosages used, the duration of the effect varies from a couple of months to several months.

The action of the drug slowly decreases over time as the affected axons sprout new nerve terminals which continually restore the impaired transmission. During this phase the damaged synapse itself will regenerate its function (de Paiva et al. 1999).

> Botulinum toxin only acts after ingestion or injection. Topical application is insufficient.
> Claims of creams that induce botulinum toxin A effects have to be questioned.

## 1.4 Antidote

Although a BNT antidote exists, it is unable to reverse any drug effects that have arisen. Once symptoms become visible, the toxin has already bound to the synapse and the late application of antibodies has no effects. Please note that antibodies are nevertheless quite helpful in botulism occurring after accidental ingestion of contaminated foods when BNT might still diffuse in the body from the gastrointestinal tract.

## 1.5 Different Products

So far, there are several BNT-A products and one BNT-B product on the market.

The BNT-A products differ in their amount of protein as well as in the amount of albumin added (Table 1.1). At the moment Botox, also marketed in some countries as Botox Aesthetic/Vistabel/Vistabex for aesthetic indications, and Dysport share the majority of the aesthetic market. The new German BNT-A preparation Xeomin is only available in a few countries so far, and lacks clinical data on its efficacy in aesthetic medicine. NeuroBloc (also marketed as Myobloc) is the only commercially available type B BNT. Although there is some data on its efficacy in aesthetic indications, it is not often used for these indications (Baumann et al. 2003).

> Botox may be marketed as Botox Aesthetics, Vistabel or Vistabex. For simplification in this book we will talk only about Botox when referring to dosages.

## 1.6 Units of Botulinum Toxin

The concept of calculating the dosage units for the different products Botox and Dysport is not easy to understand and may not be necessary. The user must only be aware that the dosage units of different products do not relate to each other. There are some attempts to offer ratios for these products. However, apart from one trial with severe methodological shortcomings (Lowe et al. 2005) there are no comparative clinical trials for aesthetic indications. For Botox and Dysport, based on the available data from placebo controlled clinical trials and dosages recommended at consensus conferences, the ratio is close to 1:2.5 – 1:3. The manufacturer claims that Xeomin has a 1:1 ratio to Botox. However, we have little experience and no published data on aesthetic indications for this BTN-A formulation so far to support this claim (Table 1.1).

Therefore, when in doubt, instead of using ratios we would recommend the treating physician to go back to the data from clinical trials or consensus conferences.

> Do not get confused by units or ratios between different products. In case of doubt one should go back to the clinical trial data or data from consensus conferences.

In this book the dosages recommended are the dosages that in our experience have the best effect in the majority of patients. For some indications these recommended dosages are based on clinical trials. However, for most indications no clinical trials have been performed so far.

## 1.7  Off-Label Use

Botox and Dysport are not licensed for aesthetic indications in all countries. In addition, the license is usually limited to the glabella area. In cases where no labelling or a limited labelling exists, the physician has to deal with off-label use. The patient must be informed if the product is used for an off-label indication.

As is sometimes the case with licensing of an other indication, the drug name is changed: basically the same brand may be available for off-label as well as labelled use. For example, in Germany Botox is listed for various neurological indications but not for aesthetic indications. However, for the treatment of the glabella area, the same drug is available as Vistabel. Both drugs contain exactly the same BNT, but Botox comes in 100 U vials and Vistabel in 50 U vials.

All the companies are trying to obtain licenses for aesthetic indications, therefore, it seems quite likely that the number of countries where the major aesthetic indications are still off-label will decrease over time. Nevertheless, it is also clear that for the present time in most countries only some indications will be licensed, such as the treatment of the glabella.

> Do not worry too much about off-label use. For Botox and Dysport there are enough studies proving efficacy and safety. The patient, however, must be informed when the product is used for an off-label indication.

## 1.8  New Drugs

At the moment several companies are working on new BNT preparations. These new products should be carefully evaluated and compared with the products presently on the market. It is always important to consider the evidence behind these new drugs. Randomized controlled clinical trials based on aesthetic indications should be the gold standard which new BNT preparations have to match. A '*This brand of botulinum toxin is comparable or even better than that brand of botulinum toxin!*' without good supporting data is not enough.

## 1.9  Evidence Behind the Use of BNT-A

In contrast to injectable fillers, the evidence behind the use of BNT-A in aesthetic medicine is much larger – at least for the two leading brands Botox and Dysport.

In the following chapter the evidence for the efficacy and safety of the different BNT-A preparations will be discussed for some key questions. In order to reduce bias only large studies, e.g. only studies of more than 50 patients will be included in this review.

## 1.10 Efficacy: Optimal Dosage

**Key question 1:** *What is the optimal dosage for treating the glabella?*

This is an important question. The glabella is probably the most frequently treated area. Fortunately there are several clinical trials available that try to answer this question. The question will be discussed for both brands separately.

What should efficacy measure? BNT targets the activity of the mimic muscles. Therefore, the ability of the toxin to reduce muscular movements should be measured. Usually it is not the muscular strength itself, but the effect of the reduction of muscular strength on the severity of wrinkles, which is measured by clinical scales. In most clinical trials four-point rating scales (with 0 for no and 3 for severe wrinkles) have been used to measure efficacy (Honeck et al. 2003).

In addition, subjective improvement is an important outcome measure. Here several scales have been used.

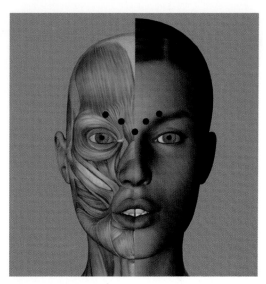

**Fig. 1.1.** Injection points as in the early Botox-Glabella studies (based on Carruthers et al. 2002)

### 1.10.1 Botox

There are several trials focusing on the optimal dosage of Botox in the area of the glabella. The standard dosage used is 20 Botox U. In the first large placebo-controlled trial, patients with moderate to severe glabellar lines at maximum frown received intramuscular injections of 20 U BNT-A or placebo into five glabellar sites (Fig. 1.1). A total of 264 patients were enrolled (203 treated with BNT-A, 61 with placebo). There was a significantly greater reduction in glabellar line severity with BTX-A than with placebo (all measures, every follow-up visit; P < 0.022). The effect was maintained for many patients throughout 120 days (Carruthers et al. 2002).

The same authors investigated in a double-blind, randomized clinical trial the efficacy, safety and duration of the effect of four dosages of BNT type A in the treatment of glabellar rhytids in females. Eighty female subjects with moderate to severe wrinkles at maximum frown entered the study. Patients were randomly administered 10, 20, 30 or 40 Botox U in seven injection points (Fig. 1.2). Objectively, 10 U of BNT type A was significantly less effective than 20, 30 or 40 U. The relapse rate at 4 months was significantly higher in the 10-U group (83%) versus 40, 30 or 20 U (28%, 30% and 33% respectively). The authors concluded that 20–40 Botox U was significantly more effective at reducing glabellar lines than 10 U (Carruthers et al. 2005).

A similar study in male patients was published the same year. In this comparable study, 80 men were randomized to receive a total dose of either 20, 40, 60 or 80 U of Botox distributed in seven points in the glabellar and lower forehead area. The 40, 60 and 80 U dosages of BNT type A were consistently more effective in reducing glabellar lines than the 20-U dose (duration, peak response rate, improvement from baseline). There was a dose-dependent increase in both the response rate at maximum frown and the duration of effect assessed by the trained observer.

1

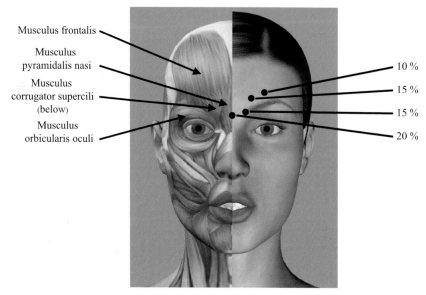

Musculus frontalis

Musculus
pyramidalis nasi

Musculus
corrugator supercili
(below)

Musculus
orbicularis oculi

10 %

15 %

15 %

20 %

**Fig. 1.2.** Injection points as in the recent Botox-Glabella studies (based on Carruthers et al. 2005)

The authors conclude that male participants with glabellar rhytids benefit from starting dosages of at least 40 U of Botox (Carruthers et al. 2005).

Based on these studies, the recommended Botox dosage for the glabella should be at least 20 Botox U. Men might benefit from even higher dosages starting with 40 Botox U.

### 1.10.2  Dysport

So far there have been three trials published focusing on the optimal dosage for the glabella (Ascher et al. 2004, Ascher et al. 2005, Rzany et al. 2006). The first study from Asher et al. (2004) is a dose-ranging study comparing 25, 50 and 75 Dysport U with placebo. A total of 119 patients with moderate to severe glabellar lines at rest were treated. The dosage was distributed over five intramuscular glabellar sites forming a bird-shaped pattern (Fig. 1.1). Outcome measures included evaluations of glabellar lines by independent experts from blinded standardized photographs at rest 1 month after treatment, physician evaluations and patient assessments

during a 6-month period. A significant efficacy was reported for the three BNT-A groups for at least 3 months after injection (at least P <.015). Investigator and patient evaluations suggested that 50 U was the optimal dosage (Ascher et al. 2004).

**Answer to key question 1:** The initial doses focused on 20 Botox U for the glabella. In two subsequent studies higher doses were recommended. However, different injection points were used. The latter studies included two additional points targeting not only the corrugator but also parts of the frontalis muscle. For Dysport the recommended dose for the glabella is 50 Dysport U. Based on these studies, a ratio for Botox and Dysport of 1:2.5 seams reasonable.

### 1.11  Effectiveness: Dosages and Repeated Treatments

**Key question 2:** *How often do patients come back and does the required dosage change after frequent visits?*

This is an important question. The frequency of re-injection visits depends on several factors: the regaining of muscular movement (which depends on the strength of muscles and the initial dose), the consequently increased visibility of mimic wrinkles, and other factors such as costs.

## 1.11.1  Botox

So far there has been no data published. There is, however, information from a poster that was presented during the EADV 2004 (Carruthers A and Carruthers J, 2004). In this study, data from a 50-patient cohort was investigated. Patients needed to have at least ten treatments. The glabella was the most frequently treated area. No specific dosage for the glabella is given. The mean dosage for all areas treated was 40 Botox U. The median interval between treatments was 17.1 weeks with a range from 0.43 to 155.3 weeks.

## 1.11.2  Dysport

In the German-Austrian retrospective study, 945 patients were followed for at least three consecutive injections. The median interval between BNT-A treatment cycles was 5.9-6.5 months (25th–75th percentile: 4.4–8.9 months) and changed little with repeated treatments (Fig. 2.2).

For the glabella the median BNT-A dosage over all treatment cycles in those who received injections in the glabella was 50–60 Dysport U (25th–75th percentile: 40–70 U); for those who received injections in the glabella only, the median BNT-A dosage was 50–70 Dysport U (25th–75th percentile: 50–100 U) The dosage did not change over the different study periods. (Rzany et al. 2007).

**Answer to key question 2:** There are two patient cohorts. Based on these data, patients treated with Botox returned three times a year, patients treated with Dysport twice a year for re-injection.

## 1.12  Safety

Here it is important not only to consider short-term safety but also long-term safety. Short-term safety is affected by the proportion of patients in whom muscles adjacent to the treated areas are influenced. For the glabella area this means the number of patients who will develop eyelid ptosis after injection with BNT-A. Again, it is the clinical trials that count.

## 1.13  Short-term Safety: Eyelid Ptosis

Short-term safety will be measured by clinical trials.

**Key question 3:** *How many patients developed eyelid ptosis after treatment of the glabella?*

## 1.13.1  Botox

Using Botox in the glabellar area, Carruthers et al. reported a lid ptosis rate of 5.4% in their first large placebo-controlled study (6 out of 203 patients; Carruthers et al. 2002), declining to 1.0% (2 out of 202 patients) in a subsequent study (Carruthers et al. 2003). In the most recent studies no lid ptosis occurred in a study of 160 patients (Carruthers et al. 2005; Carruthers and Carruthers 2005).

## 1.13.2  Dysport

When using Dysport, Ascher et al. reported no ptosis in his 102 patients treated with 25, 50 and 75 U (Ascher et al. 2004). In the German study, only one case of eyelid ptosis was reported among

1

127 patients treated with 50 Dysport U (Rzany et al. 2006).

**Answer to key question 3:** The risk for eyelid ptosis is present. However, it is small and temporary.

## 1.14  Long-term Safety: Eyelid Ptosis

Long-term safety will usually not be investigated by clinical trials. Here patient cohorts will be able to answer the questions. Fortunately, we have data from two large cohorts for the two major brands.

**Key question 4:** *What is the risk for eyelid ptosis after repeated treatments?*

### 1.14.1  Botox

In the Carruthers study (Carruthers and Carruthers 2004), adverse events were documented in 5 (0.6%) of 853 treatments. Eyelid ptosis was reported three times.

### 1.14.2  Dysport

In the German/Austrian retrospective study, adverse events (AE) were, in general, uncommon. Of the 945 patients, 90.6% (n = 856) did not experience any AE over any treatment cycle. The total AE rate per treatment cycle was 4.1% (n = 39/945) in cycle one, decreasing to 2.0% (n = 11/553) in cycle five, giving an overall mean incidence of 2.5% per treatment cycle. Importantly, most AEs were mild and resolved without further intervention. There were no serious or unexpected AEs.

Local hematoma was the most frequently reported AE (1.25% per treatment cycle; range: 1.8–0.7%). Lid or brow ptosis was uncommon (0.46% of treatment cycles; range: 0.85–0.1%) and

generally mild. All patients who experienced lid or brow ptosis (n = 16) received injections to the glabella or frontalis. A total of 3698 treatments in the glabella or frontalis were given to 907 patients. Therefore, the incidence of lid or brow ptosis in patients who received injections to the glabella and/or frontalis regions was 0.51% per treatment cycle or 1.8% per patient (Rzany et al. 2007).

**Answer to key question 4:** The risk for eyelid ptosis after repeated treatments is very small.

Please note that further information on safety is available in Chapter 7.

## 1.15  Marketing and Evidence

The market for BNT-A in aesthetic medicine is still growing. However, as in every market, there is close competition between companies. Therefore, it is important to keep a clear mind when a company claims superiority in efficacy and safety for their product. The following questions might come in handy when being approached by a representative of the company with new data claiming to show either better efficacy or safety.

*What dosages and dilutions were used?* This is very important: if you compare two products, one with a higher and one with a lower dosage, it might not be a surprise that the product with a relatively higher dose has more side effects.

*How good is the clinical trial?* It is not necessary to be a specialist of evidence based medicine (EBM). Just keep the following questions in mind when looking at a clinical trial.

*Was the trial randomized?* i.e. were the treatment groups distributed by chance? If not, just disregard it.

*Was the trial blinded?* Good clinical trials should always be blinded. A good example of a possibly absolute blinding is an expert committee who grades efficacy based on photographs.

*Were the treatment groups equal after randomization?* Sometimes randomization might fail. If there are differences in gender or age between the study groups, be extremely cautious when looking at the data. In such a case, the analysis should be at least multivariate to try to account for the failure of randomization. Do not worry about the statistical test! Just look to see whether the analysis was uni– or multivariate. If the analysis was univariate (e.g. comparing only one factor at a time) it could be prone to more biases than a multivariate analysis.

*How big was the trial?* If you have a trial which assesses the superiority or inferiority of two BNT preparations, the number of patients should be high since only small differences are likely. So if a head-to-head trial has less than 100 patients it might be better to disregard it.

> What should a good clinical trial be?
> Randomized, blinded, large enough to answer the question!

## 1.16   References

Ascher B et al. (2004) A multicenter, randomized, double-blind, placebo-controlled study of efficacy and safety of 3 doses of botulinum toxin A in the treatment of glabellar lines. J Am Acad Dermatol 51(2):223–33

Baumann L et al. (2003) A double-blinded, randomized, placebo-controlled pilot study of the safety and efficacy of Myobloc (botulinum toxin type B)-purified neurotoxin complex for the treatment of crow's feet: a double-blinded, placebo-controlled trial. Dermatol Surg 29(5):508–15

Carruthers A, Carruthers J (2004) Long-term safety review of subjects treated with botulinum toxin A for cosmetic use. Poster at the EADV

Carruthers A, Carruthers J (2005) Prospective, double-blind, randomized, parallel-group, dose-ranging study of botulinum toxin type A in men with glabellar rhytids. Dermatol Surg 31(10):1297–303

Carruthers J et al. (2002) A multicenter, double-blind, randomized, placebo-controlled study of the efficacy and safety of botulinum toxin type A in the treatment of glabellar lines. J Am Acad Dermatol 46(6):840–9.

Carruthers A et al. (2003) A prospective, double-blind, randomized, parallel-group, dose-ranging study of botulinum toxin type A in female subjects with horizontal forehead rhytides. Dermatol Surg 29(5):461–7

Carruthers A et al. (2005) Dose-ranging study of botulinum toxin type A in the treatment of glabellar rhytids in females. Dermatol Surg 31(4):414–22; discussion 422

de Paiva A et al. (1999) Functional repair of motor end-plates after botulinum neurotoxin type A poisoning: biphasic switch of synaptic activity between nerve sprouts and their parent terminals. Proc Natl Acad Sci USA 96(6):3200–5

Dressler D (2006) [Pharmacological aspects of therapeutic botulinum toxin preparations.]. Nervenarzt 77(8):912–921

Honeck P et al. (2003) Reproducibility of a four-point clinical severity score for glabellar frown lines. Br J Dermatol 149(2):306–10

Huang W et al. (2000) Pharmacology of botulinum toxin. J Am Acad Dermatol 43(2 Pt 1):249–59

Lowe PL et al. (2005) A comparison of two botulinum type A toxin preparations for the treatment of glabellar lines: double-blind, randomized, pilot study. Dermatol Surg 31(12):1651–4

Rzany B et al. (2006) Efficacy and safety of 3- and 5-injection patterns (30 and 50 U) of botulinum toxin A (Dysport) for the treatment of wrinkles in the glabella and the central forehead region. Arch Dermatol 142(3):320–6

Rzany B et al. (2007) Repeated botulinum toxin A injections for the treatment of lines in the upper face: A retrospective study of 4103 treatments in 945 patients Dermatol Surg 33 (s1), S18–S25

# Chapter 2

# Patient Selection

Mauricio de Maio, Berthold Rzany

**2**

## Contents

Not every patient is suitable for treatment with BNT. To avoid dissatisfied patients, or even adverse events, the indication for BNT treatment has to be thoroughly evaluated.

## 2.1 Indications for BNT

*Mauricio de Maio*

### 2.1.1 Introduction

The aging process is a sum of genetic and environmental influences. Intrinsic aging is mainly represented by chronological processes and leads to atrophy with skin excess and laxity, eye bags and the presence of gravitational folds (Fig. 2.1). The most effective treatment here might be surgery with muscle repositioning and skin and eye bags excess removal. Extrinsic aging is mainly caused by photo-damage which harms the skin – epidermis and dermis – leading to static wrinkles, dryness and aging spots (Fig. 2.2). The treatment of environmental aging is mainly conducted through lasers, peels, bleaching agents, fillers and botulinum toxin.

Mimic wrinkles are signs of expressed emotions. The expression of emotions is fundamental to communication between humans. Unintentional projection of emotions, due to abnormal muscular behavior, may be an impediment to accurate communication and understanding. If

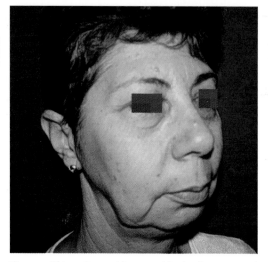

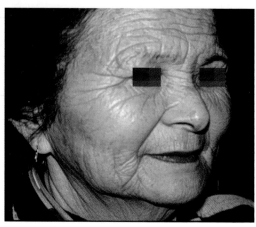

**Fig. 2.1.** This patient, with saggy skin, jowls, upper and lower eyelid skin excess and eye bags, is a typical surgical candidate. The use of BNT-A in this case would only give suboptimal results

**Fig. 2.2.** This patient with asiatic skin with deep static wrinkles in dynamic areas presents a complex pattern for treatment. The single use of BNT-A in this patient will lead to frustrating results

someone projects anger or sadness, even though he is perfectly happy, he will be misunderstood (Fig. 2.3).

Experience has changed the way botulinum toxin is now used. Not only has the technique changed but so has the dose to be injected in specific areas. Patients' feedback after the injections and the analyses of results has led to the understanding that muscular inhibition does not necessarily promote a cosmetic upgrade. The feared 'frozen look' belongs to the past and both patients and injectors understand that a natural look is desired. There are some stigmatized signs that should be avoided.

The duration of effect is now the current issue. Patients do not understand why injections may last seven months in some and only two in others! Patients are different and so is muscular behavior. Many injectors do not individualize the treatment, and also may not understand why some patients have such a short duration of effect when using standard doses. Some of the patients are symmetrical while others are quite asymmetrical (Figs. 2.4 and 2.5). Other patients have single muscle insertions while others may have multiple muscle insertions, which may also

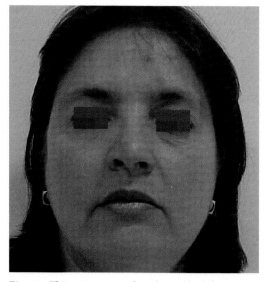

**Fig. 2.3.** This patient, even though a perfectly happy person, always looks sad due to deep marionette lines

vary the choice of the injection site (Figs. 2.6 and 2.7).

Before treatment, the muscular pattern must be evaluated. Patients may be divided into three groups before treatment, based on their muscles tonus: kinetic, hyperkinetic and hypertonic. De-

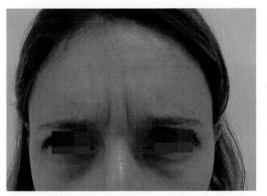

**Fig. 2.4.** This patient is quite symmetrical and injection sites should also obey this symmetry

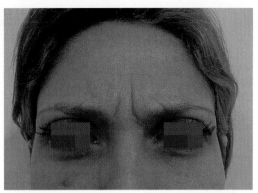

**Fig. 2.5.** This patient has a stronger corrugator on her left. Note that the dose cannot be the same for both sides in this patient

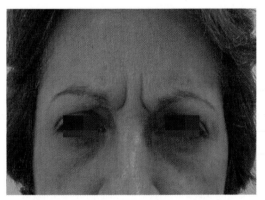

**Fig. 2.6.** The distribution of the injection sites should be undertaken according to muscle insertion. This patient has a single corrugator insertion

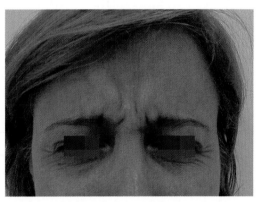

**Fig. 2.7.** In contrast to Fig. 2.6, this patient has multiple corrugator fiber insertions along the eyebrow. Dissatisfaction with BNT-A treatment is not unusual if the injection sites and dosages are not adapted for each situation

pending on the area to be treated, there will be a dominant characteristic. Patients may be hyperkinetic in one area and hypokinetic in another, so the dose should be given according to the muscular pattern of each patient.

## 2.1.2 Kinetic Patients

The kinetic patient's expression is "I move my muscles when I want". There is a concordance of emotion and mimetic expression. If the patient wants to express surprise while talking, for example, the m. frontalis is contracted and the eyebrows are raised. If the patient wants to express anger or concern, the muscles at the glabella area are contracted. There is a perfect timing of the mimics and the emotional feeling. The interlocutor understands easily both what is said and what is expressed. The interlocutor's eyes deviate to the muscular contraction exactly when the emotion is expressed. In static analysis, there is no wrinkle formation at the treatment area.

The duration of effect in kinetic patients is the longest among the groups. It may last 7–9 months

2

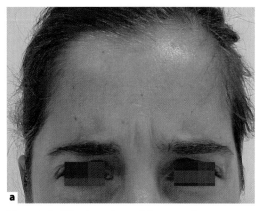
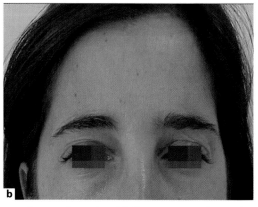

**Fig. 2.8a,b.** Kinetic patient: while expressing anger or concern, the muscles at the glabella area are not deep. After BNT-A, there are neither static nor dynamic lines. This may be considered the ideal patient with complete wrinkle removal and a long-lasting result. Please note that there is no m. procerus action in this patient, only the action of the m. corrugatores

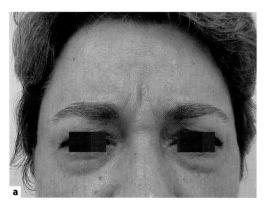
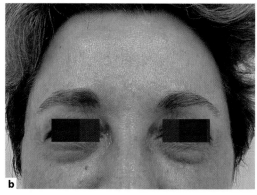

**Fig. 2.9a,b.** This is also a kinetic patient with mild muscle contraction and complete wrinkle removal after treatment with BNT-A. Note that this patient presents both m. corrugatores and m. procerus actions. This means that the injection sites should be different compared with Fig. 2.8a,b

and sometimes even longer. The procedure is usually undertaken only once a year. They are ideal candidates for treatment. Both cosmetic practitioners and patients are very satisfied with the procedure. There is absolutely no line formation after the injection of BNT-A. However, some patients may present only corrugator contraction (Figs. 2.8), while others may present both corrugator and procerus contraction (Figs. 2.9). The choice of injection sites should be adapted for each case.

Kinetic patients are known by the phrase: "I express my emotion when I want". The duration of effect is the longest out of all groups.

### 2.1.3 Hyperkinetic Patients

In this group, patients have no concordance between muscular contraction and the emotion to be expressed. In general, the muscle cycles more

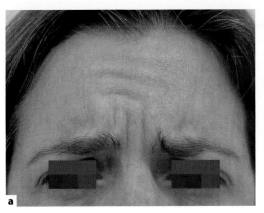 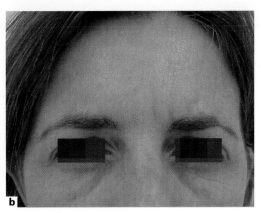

**Fig. 2.10a,b.** Hyperkinetic patients have stronger muscles and the result after the first injection can be almost complete removal of wrinkles. However, they normally need repeated doses or higher doses to obtain perfect results. After treatment the patient still presents some muscle contraction at the glabella area that may be reinjected with BNT-A to obtain optimal results

rapidly than the desired emotion or the contraction may appear without the willing of emotional expression. For example, a speaker is doing a presentation in front of an audience and is talking slowly and the muscles in the forehead move without the desire of expressing surprise or even concern. The m. frontalis and the m. corrugator contract in repeated cycles independently and excessively. The interlocutor, instead of paying attention to what is said, keeps his eyes fixed on the mimics. Hyperkinetic patients are victims of their muscular contraction: the muscle contracts involuntarily during speech and/or at a faster rate, not necessarily expressing the emotion of preoccupation or angriness, pertinent to the glabella area, for example. Vertical and/or horizontal dynamic lines are of a moderate degree but are not present at static positions. For these patients, the results may last from 4–6 months, sometimes even less. Patients return for treatment twice or three times a year. This is the most common group for BNT-treatment. Patients and injectors are pleased with the result although the former may wish it could last a little bit longer. When the effect starts to fade, they quickly come back for another injection. It is quite common for these patients to come back for an extra dose to improve the results (Fig. 2.10a,b).

> Hyperkinetic patients are victims of excessive muscular contraction. In general, they do not wait for total muscular recovery to get another shot.

### 2.1.4 Hypertonic Patients

Hypertonic patients are the negative result of lack of control of hyperkinetic patients. Their sentence is "I cannot relax" and get disappointed when asked "Are you angry?" In fact, they are happy, have slept well and their life is at its best. Their emotion is completely contaminated by the inability of specific muscles to relax. How can someone express lightness when the m. corrugator and m. procerus do not relax? How can they prove they are not angry or concerned when the mimics demonstrate exactly these emotions? For these people, immediate acceptance by others hardly ever happens. Even to themselves, looking in the mirror each morning and seeing the m. depressor anguli oris over-contracted and the oral commissure falling down, expressing sadness and tiredness, is not encouraging. They are the group that particularly needs treatment and usually gets frustrated with it. The duration of re-

2

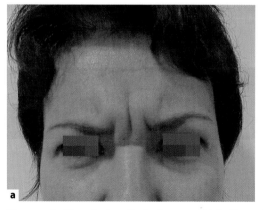
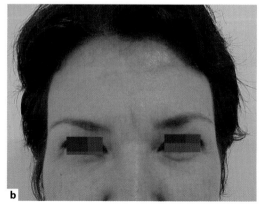

**Fig. 2.11a,b.** Hypertonic patient: after correct injection and the use of an extra dose there is still a vertical line at the glabella area. This patient was advised before the BNT-A treatment that the additional use of an injectable filler would be necessary

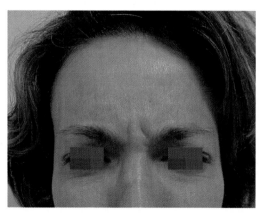

**Fig. 2.12.** This kinetic patient presents a mild contraction on her left and mild asymmetry

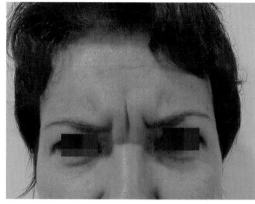

**Fig. 2.13.** In contrast, this hypertonic patient presents very strong corrugators and procerus. The single use of BNT-A will not be able to provide complete reshape of the glabella area in this kind of hypertonic patient. Fillers should also be offered

sult in these patients is the shortest of all groups. Both patients and practitioners get disappointed with the injection for two main reasons: the wrinkle does not disappear completely and muscular contraction may be blocked for only 1 or 2 months. The disappointment comes from the fact that the same results as for the kinetic and hyperkinetic patients are expected. In this special group the target is to inhibit hypertonicity and relax the muscle. The hypertonic patient

should become hyperkinetic and finally kinetic. To achieve this, it is not uncommon for the patient to undergo four or five treatments a year! In addition, fillers should be used to achieve better overall results (Fig. 2.11a,b). It is easier to understand the limitation of treatments when we compare kinetic and hypertonic patients (Figs. 2.12 and 2.13).

> Both hypertonic patients and injectors get disappointed with the result. They may require four or five treatments a year!

## 2.1.5 Outcome Analysis

When botulinum toxin started to be used for cosmetic purposes, one of the main complaints from patients was about the 'frozen look'. These times should be gone. Based on muscular behavior after the injection, patients can also be divided into three groups: atonic, hypotonic and hypokinetic.

When critically analyzing the result of the botulinum toxin injection, we should be able to have balanced the areas where we wanted a complete absence of movement but maintenance of position, and where a slight movement is desired. The resulting hypokinesis seems to be the most desired effect for many areas in the face. The decrease in muscle cycles and the slowdown of muscle excursion is one the most important aspects that leads to a natural look. However, patients must understand that some initial movement does not mean loss of effect and they must be told so before the treatment.

> The resulting hypokinesis is the ideal muscular pattern after the treatment for promoting a natural look.

Excessive blocking of specific muscles may lead to an unpleasant appearance. There are muscles that should have the minimal tonus preserved in order to maintain the anatomic structure at its right position. For instance, the m. frontalis, besides elevating the eyebrows, is also responsible for maintaining them at their correct level. If the m. frontalis is over-injected, the minimal tonus is blocked and as a consequence, the brow or pseudo ptosis may result. What is a natural look then?

It depends! Injectors should initially analyze the muscular pattern, adaptation behavior and what would promote a cosmetic upgrade for the patient. If we didactically divide the face into three thirds, we have to try to make them harmonious among themselves. Botulinum toxin is a powerful agent for the upper third: it can erase wrinkles, lift the eyebrows and improve the eye contour. If the patient presents severe photo-damage, the skin of the three thirds is compromised and what can be improved in the skin appearance in the upper third, can barely be achieved in the lower and even less in the mid third. The question that should be asked now is: Is it reasonable to give a full treatment in the upper third while the mid and lower thirds cannot achieve the same performance? Botulinum toxin treatments were carried out like this previously, and this may be one of the main reasons that it frightened many patients.

Not only should we avoid complete blocking in some areas, but we should also analyze whether partial blocking is still too excessive.

> A natural look implies not only which area should be fully blocked, but also the percentage of blocking that each partial treatment must have.

When analyzing the patient to make the right decision about full and partial blocking, it is good to come back and review what happens in the aging process. Let us try to visualize a child or an adolescent. Focus on the upper third: there are no lines; the m. frontalis excursion is limited and the m. corrugator and m. procerus present do not show a very evident contraction. It is more common to see the surprise on their faces than to see the angriness at the glabella level. If we analyze the face, we will notice that the elevators are more important than the depressors in youth. With aging process, this behavior changes and the depressors start to play an important role, causing a tired and sad look. Botulinum

2

toxin should be used to block the depressors and give the patients a more refreshed look.

> With aging the depressors become stronger than the elevators, leading to a tired and sad appearance. Botulinum toxin should be used to promote a more refreshed look.

### 2.1.6  Tips and Tricks

■ The ideal patients to start with the use of botulinum toxin are the kinetic ones. Hyperkinetics are those who will particularly need our assistance and will return more often for retreatment in our offices. Hypertonic patients should be told immediately about the limitations of treatment with BNT-A alone and should be treated with fillers or other surgical methods, such as subcision or direct excision with suture.

### 2.1.7  References

Becker-Wegerich P, Rauch L, Ruzicka T. (2001) Botulinum toxin A in the therapy of mimic facial lines. Clin Exp Dermatol. 26(7):619–30. Review

Ellis DA, Tan AK (1997) Cosmetic upper-facial rejuvenation with botulinum toxin. J Otolaryngol. 26(2):92–6

Manaloto RM, Alster TS (1999) Periorbital rejuvenation: a review of dermatologic treatments. Dermatol Surg. 25(1):1–9. Review

Mendez-Eastman SK (2003) BOTOX: A review. Plast Surg Nurs. 23(2):64–9

Pribitkin EA, Greco TM, Goode RL, Keane WM (1997) Patient selection in the treatment of glabellar wrinkles with botulinum toxin type A injection. Arch Otolaryngol Head Neck Surg. 123(3):321–6

Robb-Nicholson C (2002) By the way doctor. I've been reading about the cosmetic benefits of Botox injections, but what are the risks? Harv Womens Health Watch. 10(3):8

Sclafani AP, Kwak E (2005) Alternative management of the aging jaw line and neck. Facial Plast Surg. 21(1):47–54

## 2.2  Contraindications for Botulinum Toxin

*Berthold Rzany*

To avoid adverse events certain contraindications have to be ruled out prior to the treatment with BNT.

### 2.2.1  General Contraindications

#### 2.2.1.1  Dysmorphism

Dysmorphic patients are those obsessively preoccupied with real or imaginary defects. They take great measures to point out defects which are not viewed by the physician. In general, those defects are minor but are perceived by them to be disfiguring. The inability to deal with unavoidable scars is also a warning that dissatisfaction may rise after the cosmetic procedure. Some patients do have a real psychiatric or emotional disorder. Patients with borderline personality, obsessive-compulsive and narcissistic disorders should be avoided.

Here it is at the discretion of the aesthetic physician to tell the patient in a very compassionate way that the result they are looking for cannot be obtained by this procedure.

### 2.2.2  Drug specific Contraindications

#### 2.2.2.1  Diseases with Pathological Neuromuscular Transmission

BNT treatment is contraindicated in patients with amyotrophic lateral sclerosis, myasthenia gravis, multiple sclerosis and Eaton Lambert syndrome since all these conditions show pathological neuromuscular transmission, which may worsen by systemic BNT effects. In fact Cote et al (Cote et al. 2005) report a case of aggravated Myasthenia gravis after the injection of BNT. As with every other drug too an absolute contraindication would be a known hypersensitivity or allergy to the BNT-class or its excipients (Vartanian et al. 2005).

No reliable data about teratogenic effects of BTN in humans has been published so far. Although no complications in accidental pregnancies have been reported so far, BNT treatment of pregnant women and nursing mothers should not be performed.

### 2.2.2.2 Drug Interactions

For the usage of BNT in aesthetic medicine there have been no reports of clinically significant drug-drug interactions so far, yet one should consider possible interactions with drugs that interfere with neuromuscular or neuroglandular transmission. These substances include aminoglycosides, cyclosporine, d-penicillamine, depolarizing and non-depolarizing muscle relaxants, quinidine, magnesium sulfate, lincosamides and aminoquinolones. While most of these substances potentiate the BNT-effect, aminoquinolones and chloroquine can inhibit its activity (Simpson 1982).

### 2.2.2.3 Injection related Contraindications

BNT is injected. Therefore, any bleeding disorder even when using very small needles has an increased risk of bruising. The use of drugs interfering the bleeding time is usually with these superficial injections not an absolute contraindication. Patients for example on acetylic acid should be advised that there is an increased risk of bruising related to the injections but may be treated.

### 2.2.3 References

Adamson PA, Kraus WM.(1995) Management of patient dissatisfaction with cosmetic surgery. Fac Plast Surg 11:99–104

Baker TJ (1978) Patient selection and psychological evaluation. Clin Plast Surg 5:3–14

Cote TR, Mohan AK et al. (2005). Botulinum toxin type A injections: adverse events reported to the US Food and Drug Administration in therapeutic and cosmetic cases J Am Acad Dermatol 53(3): 407–15

Lewis CM, Lavell S, Simpson MF (1983) Patient selection and patient satisfaction. Clin Plast Surg 1983 321–332

Katez P (1991) The dissatisfied patient. Plast Surg Nurs 11:13–16

Sarwar D (1997) The 'obsessive' cosmetic surgery patient: a consideration of body image dissatisfaction and body dysmorphic disorder. Plast Surg Nurs 17:193–197, 209

Simpson LL (1982) The interaction between aminoquinolines and presynaptically acting neurotoxins. J Pharmacol Exp Ther 222(1): 43–8

Vartanian AJ, Dayan SH (2005) Complications of botulinum toxin A use in facial rejuvenation. Facial Plast Surg Clin North Am 13(1): 1–10

Vuyk HD, Zijlker TD (1995) Psychosocial aspects of patient counseling and selection: a surgeon's perspective. Fac Plast Surg 11:55–60

# Chapter 3

# Requirements and Rules

Berthold Rzany

**3**

## Contents

## 3.1 Introduction

The requirements and rules are basically the same for every aesthetic procedure. The following list is not intended to give a complete overview but to give some hopefully helpful advice when treating aesthetic indications with botulinum toxin (BNT).

## 3.2 Documentation

A thorough documentation of all treatment-related data is highly recommended. Besides being useful for legal and billing reasons, thorough documentation will help to improve one's own performance and thus patients' satisfaction, too.

### 3.2.1 Chart

The patient's identification data, age, the history of relevant concomitant diseases, present relevant drug intake (e.g. the intake of acetylsalicylic acid!) and previous aesthetic procedures should be documented.

Furthermore, the procedure itself has to be documented. This can be either done as text or as text supported by figures of the areas to be treated. Here, the injection points, the injected U and/or volume should be stated.

### 3.2.2 Photograph

It is advisable to document the status of the patient before treatment. If possible, the photographs should be standardized. Standardization requires some effort, such as using a fixed setting or following standard procedures. Patients tend to forget their pre-treatment features and might assume that nothing has changed. In such a case, a photograph prior to the treatment session might help avoid unpleasant misunderstandings.

### 3.2.3 Consent

The consent of each patient should be thoroughly documented. Patients should date and sign the consent for each new indication. The consent form should be accompanied by a patient information brochure that includes all necessary information on the estimated efficacy and possible adverse events.

### 3.2.4 Treatment Plan

A treatment plan is highly recommended for every aesthetic procedure. Patients should be aware of the fact that BNT has a limited durability and three to four treatments per year might be necessary.

### 3.3 Staff

The staff have to be trained in several areas: marketing, quality control and assistance. Marketing: the staff should be aware of the aesthetic procedures offered and should be able to give some information about the use of botulinum toxin. Staff are responsible for monitoring the chart as well as ensuring that all necessary documents are available and signed by the patient if applicable.

### 3.4 Technical Requirements

### 3.4.1 Room

The room should be brightly lit. No shadows should decrease the visibility of the area to be treated.

### 3.4.2 Chair

Although all indications can be treated in an upright position, a reclining position is recommended, especially for anxious patients. For the treatment of platsymal bands patients should be in an upright position; otherwise the bands would not be visible.

### 3.4.3 Mirror

A mirror should accompany patient-doctor communication from the start. Using the mirror the doctor can ensure that both are speaking about exactly the same areas to be treated. At the end of the treatment the doctor might show the patient the injection points and explain the procedure again.

### 3.4.4 Cosmetic Marker

A cosmetic pen to mark the injection points can be quite helpful in reducing asymmetry. E.g. asymmetry might easily occur when treating the forehead. Here, the use of a cosmetic pen such as a lip liner will greatly reduce the risk of asymmetry.

### 3.4.5 Standard Setting

All tools required should be within reach (Table 3.1). A standard setting for treatment with BNT might prove to be helpful.

**Table 3.1.** Necessary tools to be arranged before treatment

| |
|---|
| Patient information and consent form |
| Documentation material for source data (electronic or conventional charts) |
| Hand mirror |
| Camera (conventional or digital) for photographic documentation |
| Topical local anesthetic (usually not needed) |
| Topical disinfectant (preferably without dye and non-alcoholic) |
| Non-sterile dressings |
| Cosmetic pen, for example a lip liner (marking the injection points may be quite helpful to ensure harmonious and symmetric results) |
| Vial with botulinum toxin, saline for dilution (if necessary), appropriate syringes and needles (30-gauge needles are a must, 32-gauge needles are great) |
| Cool packs or pre-cooled saline to soak compresses |
| Emergency kit (in case of the extremely unlikely event of an anaphylactic reaction) |

## 3.4.6 The Toxin

**Storage of Undiluted Toxin**

BNT has to be stored either in the refrigerator (Botox, Dysport) or under normal room conditions (Xeomin).

**Dilution**

All BNTs-A preparations have to be diluted with saline. Usually 2.5 ml saline is used to dilute the BNT-A when used in aesthetic indications. Some colleagues prefer lower or higher dilutions (Tables 3.2 and 3.3). The effect of a higher dilution is not clear. Based on a small study investigating one dose in two different volumes, it appears that a greater volume means greater diffusion into the adjacent muscles, giving greater efficacy, but also greater risk of adverse events. There was no follow-up on the duration of the effect in this study (Hsu et al. 2004).

> The standard dilution for Botox and Dysport is 2.5 ml.

**Storage of Diluted Toxin**

All manufacturers recommend the BNT-A to be only used for several hours after dilution. However, in clinical practice, BNT-A is often stored in the refrigerator for several days up to a couple of weeks. With increased storage time, a decrease in efficacy and increased risk of contamination is likely. However, Doris Hexsel reported not such a

**Table 3.2.** Botox: U per ml for different dilutions

| Botox 100 U in | 0.9% saline | | | | | |
|---|---|---|---|---|---|---|
| | 0.01 ml | 0.02 ml | 0.05 ml | 0.1 ml | 0.15 ml | 0.2 ml |
| 2.0 ml | 0.52 | 1 | 2.52 | 7 | | |
| 2.5 ml | 0.4 | 0.8 | 2 | 4 | | |
| 3.0 ml | 0.34 | 0.66 | 0.13 | 3.34 | 5 | |
| 4.0 ml | 0.26 | 0.5 | 1.26 | 3.5 | 3.76 | 5 |
| 4.5 ml | 0.22 | 0.44 | 1.12 | 2.22 | 3.34 | 4.44 |

**Table 3.3.** Dysport: U per ml for different dilutions (modified from Rzany et al. 2005)

| Dysport 500 U in | 0.9% saline | | | | | |
|---|---|---|---|---|---|---|
| | 0.01 ml | 0.02 ml | 0.05 ml | 0.1 ml | 0.15 ml | 0.2 ml |
| 2.0 ml | 2.6 | 5 | 12.6 | 25 | | |
| 2.5 ml | 2 | 4 | 10 | 20 | | |
| 3.0 ml | 1.7 | 3.3 | 8.3 | 16.7 | 25 | |
| 4.0 ml | 1.3 | 2.5 | 6.3 | 12.5 | 18.8 | 25 |
| 4.5 ml | 1.1 | 2.2 | 5.6 | 11.1 | 16.7 | 22.2 |

decrease while using BNT-A reconstituted up to six consecutive weeks before application (Hexsel et al. 2003).

## 3.4.7 Tips and Tricks

■ Most complaints from dissatisfied patients might be traced to insufficient communication between the doctor and the patient. This also applies to the cost related to these procedures! Patients should know from the start what they can expect and how much they have to pay.

## 3.4.8 References

Hexsel DM, De Almeida AT, Rutowitsch M, De Castro IA, Silveira VL, Gobatto DO, Zechmeister M, Mazzuco R, Zechmeister D (2003) Multicenter, double-blind study of the efficacy of injections with botulinum toxin type A reconstituted up to six consecutive weeks before application. Dermatol Surg. 29(5):523-9

Hsu TS, Dover JS, Arndt KA (2004) Effect of volume and concentration on the diffusion of botulinum exotoxin A. Arch Dermatol 140(11):1351-4

Rzany B, Fratila A, Heckmann M. (2005) 2. Expertentreffen zur Anwendung von Botulinum toxin A (Dysport®) in der Ästhetischen Dermatologie. Kosmetische Medizin 26:134-41

# Chapter 4

# Injection Technique

Berthold Rzany

**4**

## Contents

## 4.1  Introduction

Topical BNT treatment is a wish far away from realization. BNT needs to be injected to exert its action. There are basically two ways to inject BNT: the standard technique and the microinjection technique.

## 4.2  Standard Technique

The standard technique is used if target areas are well-defined and there is a minimal risk of adverse reactions. BNT in a volume of 0.05 ml or more is injected with a 30 or 32-gauge needle perpendicular or beveled into the skin. The standard technique is especially recommended for the mm. corrugatores. The periosteum should not be touched.

## 4.3  Microinjection Technique

The microinjection technique is used to administer low doses of BNT very superficially. BNT applied by microinjection technique in the crow's feet area will decrease the risk of an involuntary co-treatment of the m. zygomaticus major. The microinjection technique follows an intradermal approach. Small amounts of BNT (less than 0.025 ml) are injected approximately 1 cm apart, very superficially, in a technique comparable to

4

the intradermal skin test. Here the 32 gauge or at least a 30-gauge needle is highly recommended. If done correctly a small, sometimes whitish, papule can be seen (Fig. 4.1).

## 4.4 Other Techniques

BNT should usually not be injected by feathering techniques to avoid adverse events due to the involuntary co-treatment of adjacent muscles.

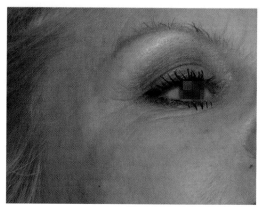

**Fig. 4.1.** Small whitish papules after applying BNT-A using the microinjection technique in the crow's feet area

# Chapter 5

# The Most Common Indications

Berthold Rzany, Mauricio de Maio

**5**

## Contents

The following chapters describe the most common indications. Although written by both authors separately, the chapters follow the same sequence and try to depict the procedures in the most 'hands on' way possible.

Please note that the doses are given in Botox and Dysport units. If you use Botox Aesthetics, Vistabel or Vistabex please keep with the Botox units.

## 5.1 Forehead

*Berthold Rzany*

### 5.1.1 Introduction

The forehead muscle is an elevator. Over treating this muscle will result in brow ptosis, which is one of the major signs of aging.

### 5.1.2 Anatomy

The venter frontalis of the m. occipitofrontalis is part of the m. epicranius. It derives from the skin of the eyebrows and glabella and intervenes with the fibres of the m. orbicularis oculi. It follows upwards where it inserts into the galea aponeurotica, the extended tendon of the m. epicranius. This muscle leads, when contracted, to the horizontal lines of the forehead. It raises the eyebrow and the upper lid and by this makes the eye look open and much bigger (Table. 5.1).

### 5.1.3 Aim of Treatment

The aim of the treatment is to decrease the forehead wrinkles.

**Table 5.1.** Overview of the muscles responsible for forehead lines

| Muscle | Action | Synergists | Antagonists |
|---|---|---|---|
| M. occipitofrontalis | Raises eyebrows, induces horizontal lines | - | M. corrugtores, m. procerus, m. depressor supercilii |

### 5.1.4 Patient Selection

Patient selection is quite straightforward. Kinetic patients are those that may present the best result: complete static and dynamic line removal without or only with slight brow ptosis (Figs. 5.1–5.4). In hyperkinetic and hypertonic patients, brow ptosis is usually inevitable. Depending on the degree of brow ptosis the result might still be desirable (Figs. 5.5–5.8). In hypertonic patients with pronounced elastosis, however, brow ptosis will inevitably lead to an aesthetic disaster (Figs. 5.9 and 5.10). In hypertonic patients with a pronounced elastosis, BNT-A might be applied only to the medial part of the forehead.

Restricting the injections to the medial fibers may lead to an undesired wrinkling just above the lateral part of the eyebrow, the so-called mephisto look. The mephisto look results from the contraction of the lateral frontalis fibers in the absence of contraction of the medial fibers. It is more visible when the glabella is treated at the same time (Figs. 5.11–5.14).

Bold patients: these patients might pose a challenge, especially when a brow ptosis is already present. Restricting the treatment to the mid forehead area might give a strange-looking appearance with residual wrinkling above a wrinkle-free zone.

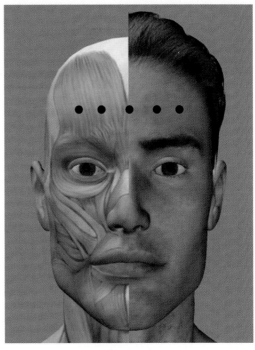

**Fig. 5.1.** Injection points targeting the central forehead area in a male kinetic patient

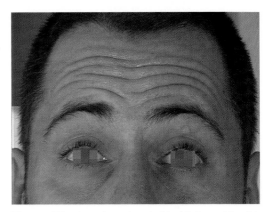

**Fig. 5.2.** Kinetic male patient in his thirties: raising his eyebrows before treatment

5

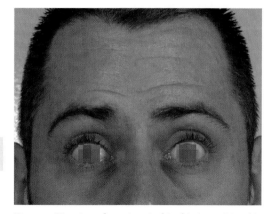

**Fig. 5.3.** Kinetic male patient in his thirties: raising his eyebrows 1 week after treatment with BNT-A

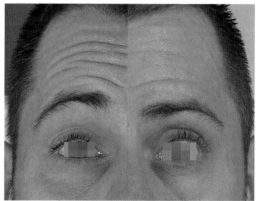

**Fig. 5.4.** Split photograph of the kinetic male patient in his thirties raising his eyebrows before and 1 week after treatment with BNT-A

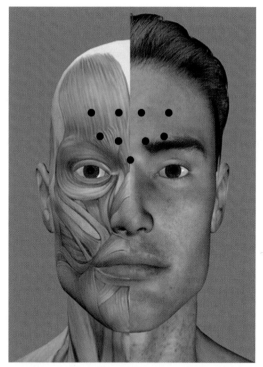

**Fig. 5.5.** Injection points targeting the central forehead area and the glabella in a male hyperkinetic patient

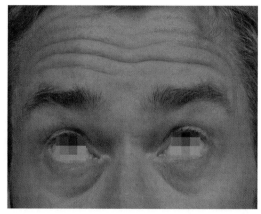

**Fig. 5.6.** Hyperkinetic male patient in his forties: raising his eyebrows before treatment

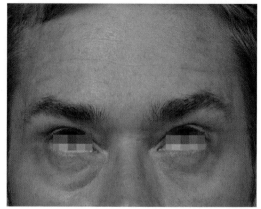

**Fig. 5.7.** Hyperkinetic male patient in his forties: raising his eyebrows 4 weeks after treatment with BNT-A

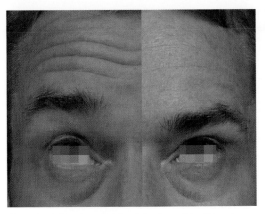

**Fig. 5.8.** Split photograph of the hyperkinetic male patient in his forties raising his eyebrows before and 4 weeks after treatment with BNT-A. Please note the slight brow ptosis

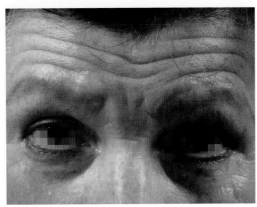

**Fig. 5.9.** Hyperkinetic/hypertonic patient in her sixties before treatment of the forehead area

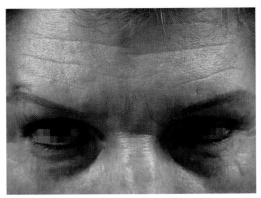

**Fig. 5.10.** Severe brow ptosis 4 weeks after treatment of the forehead area in a hyperkinetic/hypertonic patient in her sixties with BNT-A

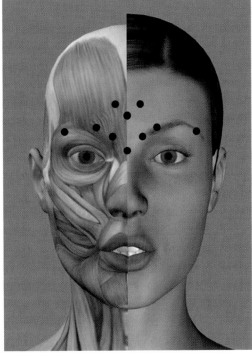

**Fig. 5.11.** Injection points targeting the central forehead area and the glabella in a hyperkinetic female patient in her early fifties

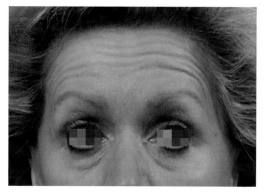

**Fig. 5.12.** Hyperkinetic patient in her early fifties: raising her eyebrows before treatment

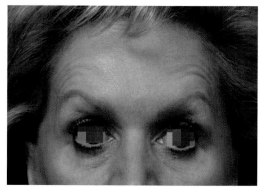

**Fig. 5.13.** Hyperkinetic patient in her early fifties: raising her eyebrows 4 weeks after treatment of the glabella, the central forehead region and a lateral brow lift. Please note the appearance of the so-called Mephisto sign

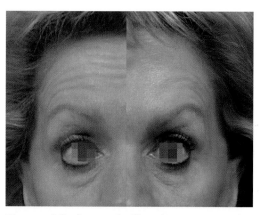

**Fig. 5.14.** Split photograph of hyperkinetic patient in her early fifties before and 4 weeks after treatment

## 5.1.5 Technique

### 5.1.5.1 Standard

Four to six injection points are sufficient to treat the forehead (Figs. 5.1, 5.5 and 5.11). The injection points should be distributed in the middle of the forehead area. If the lateral injection point is placed in the midpupillary line, the lateral parts of the m. frontalis will lift the lateral parts of the eyebrows upward (Fig. 5.11). This distribution of injection points is preferable in female patients.

In male patients the lateral injection points may be placed in a line with the lateral corner of the eye.

### 5.1.5.2 High Forehead or Wrinkle-Free Forehead

In case of a high forehead or with the treatment goal of a wrinkle-free forehead, higher doses are possible. In both cases a second line might be placed above the first line.

### 5.1.5.3 Combination with Glabella

Often the forehead is treated together with the glabella (see Chap. 5.2). In this case the total dose might be reduced to avoid a frozen expression.

Treatment of the forehead
- Four to six injection points in the middle of the forehead – the lateral points determine the degree of movement of the eyebrows (more medially placed they allow more lateral movement with an elevation of the lateral parts of the eyebrow (*female pattern*)

- Injection technique: deep, without contact with the periosteum
- Botox dose: 10–15 U total dose for one line
- Dysport dose: 25–40 U total dose for one line

doses of BNT-A (approximately 2–3 Dysport U or the equivalent of Botox) might be helpful. A low dose is mandatory to avoid brow ptosis. As a brow ptosis-free alternative, the superficial injection of an appropriate non-permanent injectable filler (e.g. hyaluronic acid or collagen) might be recommended.

## 5.1.6 Complications

### 5.1.6.1 Brow Ptosis

Brow ptosis is the most common and unwanted adverse event. It will occur in most hyperkinetic patients and in nearly all hypertonic patients. There is no correction for brow ptosis except to reassure the patient that this effect will be temporary.

### 5.1.6.2 Mephisto Sign

When restricting the forehead treatment to the area between the midpupillary lines in some patients, especially hypertonic patients, lateral movement of the m. frontalis will produce more visible wrinkles or make the existing wrinkles more visible; the so-called Mephisto sign. The Mephisto sign may be carefully corrected with an injection in the point of maximum contraction when the patient raises the forehead. The injection point should be approximately 1 cm above the orbital rim. However, be aware that this additional injection point may lead to brow ptosis.

### 5.1.6.3 Residual Upper Eyebrow Wrinkles

In some patients when the total forehead is treated some residual small wrinkles above the eyebrows may persist. Here microinjections of small

## 5.1.7 Tips and Tricks

- Listen to the patient. Make sure of what the patient wants. For a first-time treatment it might be wise to start with a minimal approach to avoid unhappy patients. Be very careful in hypertonic patients with elastosis. Here other treatment options might come first.

## 5.2 Glabella

*Berthold Rzany*

### 5.2.1 Introduction

For both the doctor and the patient, the glabella is usually the first region to be treated with BNT-A.

### 5.2.2 Anatomy

Glabellar lines are created by three muscles: the m. depressor supercilii, m. corrugator and the m. procerus. The m. depressor supercilii is the medial part of the orbicularis oculi pars orbitalis. It derives from the ligament palpebrale mediale and inserts in a fan shape cranially in the dermis of the medial part of the eyebrow. Contracting the m. depressor supercilii will draw the eyebrows down and will give this person a menacing

**Table 5.2.** Overview of the muscles responsible for glabellar lines

| Muscle | Action | Synergists | Antagonists |
| --- | --- | --- | --- |
| M. depressor supercilii | Draws medial eyebrows down | M. corrugator | M. occipitofrontalis |
| M. corrugator | Induces vertical lines | M. depressor supercilii | M. occipitofrontalis |
| M. procerus | Induces horizontal lines | M. depressor supercilii | M. occipitofrontalis |

5

expression. The m. corrugator supercilii, also seen as an independent deeper part of the orbicularis oculi pars orbitalis derives from the medial orbital ring and gradually proceeds laterally to where the muscle inserts above the middle of the eyebrow in the dermis. Contracting the m. corrugator supercilii leads to vertical lines between the eyebrows. The m. procerus originates from the bridge of the nose and inserts into to the skin of the glabella. Its fibres are interwoven with the frontalis ventral fibres of the m. occipitofrontalis. Contracting the m. procerus will induce a horizontal line between the eyebrows (Table 5.2).

### 5.2.3  Aim of Treatment

The aim of the treatment is to reduce the vertical as well as the horizontal lines of the glabella.

### 5.2.4  Patient Selection

Again, kinetic and hyperkinetic patients are best to treat. Kinetic patients only produce glabellar wrinkles if they want to denote anger or concentration and the lines are mainly superficial. Hyperkinetic patients present glabellar lines independently of willing to express anger or concentration. Lines are seen in dynamic situations and are deeper. Hypertonic patients are more difficult to treat (Figs. 5.60–5.62). In these patients BNT-A has only a moderate effect on

glabellar wrinkles, because they are present in a static situation. Here, usually an additional treatment with injectable fillers is necessary to obtain good results.

Men having stronger muscles usually require higher doses compared with women (Figs. 5.15–5.18).

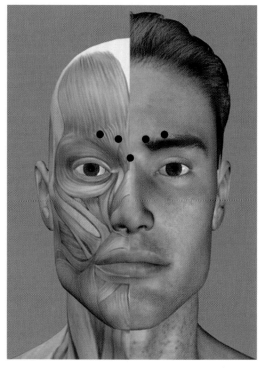

**Fig. 5.15.** Injection points targeting the glabella for male patients

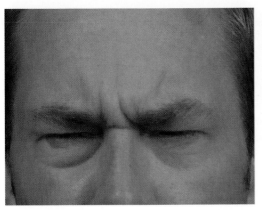

**Fig. 5.16.** Hyperkinetic/hypertonic male patient: glabella area frowning before treatment

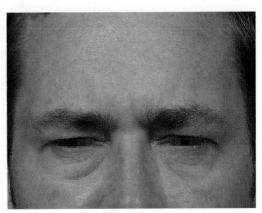

**Fig. 5.17.** Hyperkinetic/hypertonic male patient: glabella area frowning 4 weeks after treatment with BNT-A

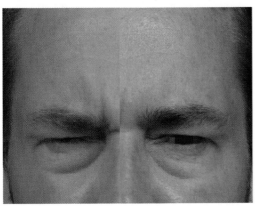

**Fig. 5.18.** Split photograph of a hyperkinetic/hypertonic male patient at rest before and 4 weeks after treatment of the glabella with BNT-A

## 5.2.5 Technique

The total dose is distributed over three to five injection points in the glabella area covering all three muscles involved in the formation of the glabellar lines.

In most patients, the first injection point is used to treat the m. procerus. The two most important points for treating the glabella are the injection points in the corrugator muscles, which are located medially about 0.5 – 1 cm above the edge of the orbital bone. Two further possible injection points are located laterally following the course of the corrugator ('swallow shaped') over these two first points. The injection should be done perpendicularly. Please take care NOT to touch the periosteum (Figs. 5.15 and 5.19).

Treatment of the glabella
- Three to five injection points
  - One point for the m. procerus (in the middle of an imaginary cross between the contralateral eyebrows and the medial corner of the eyelid)
  - One point per m. corrugator (0.5–1 cm above the medial orbital rim in extension of the exit of the n. supraorbitalis)
  - Two additional more lateral points to treat the lateral parts of the mm. corrugatores and parts of the m. frontalis (approx. 1 cm above the orbital rim)
- Injection technique: deep, without contact with the periosteum
- Botox dose: 20–40 U (total dose)
- Dysport dose: 50 U with a range from 30–70 U (*total dose*)

5

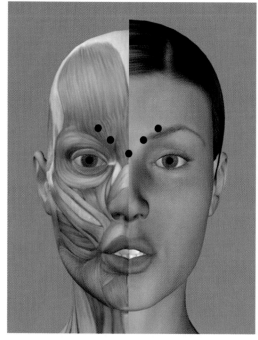

**Fig. 5.19.** Injection points targeting the glabella for female patients

## 5.2.6 Complications

### 5.2.6.1 Eyelid Ptosis

Eyelid ptosis is the effect least wanted. Eyelid ptosis occurs through the diffusion of a significant amount of toxin to the m. levator palpeprae (Fig. 5.23). Thankfully, eyelid ptosis is temporary and usually subsides after a few weeks.

### 5.2.6.2 Flattening and Broadening of the Glabella Area

Especially in hypertonic patients, the area between the medial parts of the brows is widened considerably leading to an undesirable cosmetic outcome (Figs. 5.20–5.22).

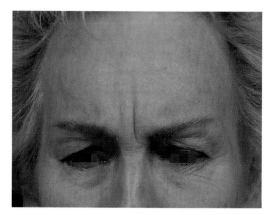

**Fig. 5.20.** Hypertonic female patient: glabella area frowning before treatment

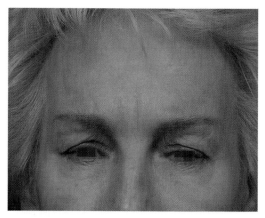

**Fig. 5.21.** Hypertonic female patient: glabella area frowning 4 weeks after treatment with BNT-A

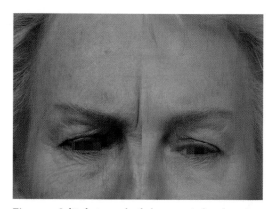

**Fig. 5.22.** Split photograph of a hypertonic female patient at rest before and 4 weeks after treatment of the glabella with BNT-A

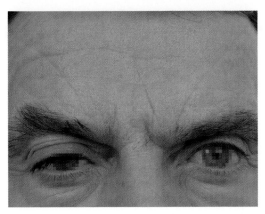

**Fig. 5.23.** Eyelid ptosis 2 weeks after injection of 50 Dysport U (hypertonic patient from the GLADYS study (Rzany et al. 2006))

### 5.2.7 Tips and Tricks

- Three injection points might not be enough in patients with a strong corrugator. Here, treating only the middle part of the corrugator might lead to residual muscular movements of the middle and lateral parts of the corrugator.
- When targeting the medial parts of the mm. corrugatores, small arterial vessels might be accidentally injured. Usually pre- and postinjection cooling helps to reduce unwanted hematoma.

## 5.3 Brow lift

*Mauricio de Maio*

### 5.3.1 Introduction

In the upper third of the face, the aging process causes gradual descent of the forehead and brow, especially its lateral third. Eyebrow mal-positioning may lead to upper eyelid fullness that may be targeted insufficiently by blepharoplasty alone.

In addition, hyperactivity of the central brow musculature may be quite common. The frontalis muscle attempts to maintain brow positioning by over-contracting its fibers and as a result produces transverse forehead creases.

Eyebrow position differs between men and women. In women, the eyebrow is ideally positioned above the supraorbital rim, while in men, it lies at the rim. The medial and lateral ends of the eyebrow should lie at the same horizontal level. Patients usually complain of a tired look and upper-eyelid fullness when these parameters are lost and especially when the lateral part of the eyebrow droops.

Many methods have been described for eyebrow lifting; however, apart from the use of injectable fillers, the majority of them are quite invasive. The most common treatments include coronal incision, pre-trichial approach, endoscopic suspensions and surgical threads. All of them need some kind of anesthesia and almost all of them need hospitalization. The use of botulinum toxin has changed the approach to eyebrow lifting, so that it is probably the most commonly used procedure of all.

### 5.3.2 Anatomy

The facial upper third extends from the hairline to the top of the eyebrows. In men with receding hairlines, the upper part of the forehead equals the superior aspect of the frontalis muscle. Its normal resting tension is responsible for the normal position of the eyebrows. The epicranial aponeurosis or galea aponeurotica covers the skull, just beneath the fat. The m. frontalis is the anterior part of the occipitofrontalis muscle. In front of the coronal suture, the aponeurosis gives origin to and is partly hidden by the frontalis bellies, which descend without any bony attachment to blend with the m. orbicularis oculi. The medial fibers of the m. frontalis blend with the m. procerus fibers and become contiguous at the nasal level. The m. frontalis has two halves and in the superior aspect of the midline forehead there is no muscle, but a fascial band.

The usual action of the m. frontalis is to raise the eyebrows in the expression of surprise and even higher with fright, and to furrow the forehead with transverse lines with thought. The eyebrows have one elevator and three opponents as depressors: the m. corrugator, the m. procerus and the m. orbicularis oculi. The m. frontalis interdigitates with the orbital m. orbicularis oculi at the nasal level. It also blends with the obliquely oriented fibers of the m. corrugator supercilli. The corrugator is a small narrow muscle that arises from the inner extremity of the superior ciliary ridge and inserts into the deep surfaces of the skin above and between the orbital rims. It lies beneath the m. frontalis and m. orbicularis oculi. The corrugator draws the eyebrows downward and inward, producing the vertical wrinkles in the glabella. It is used to squint and protect the eyes. The m. procerus originates from the nasal bone and inserts into the skin of the forehead between the eyebrows. It pulls down the medial aspect of the eyebrow and produces the horizontal line at this level. The m. orbicularis oculi when contracted pulls the complete eyebrow downwards. (Table 5.3)

## 5.3.3 Aim of Treatment

The aim of the treatment is to lift the lateral eyebrow. The medial aspect can also be lifted in selected cases. With brow lifting, patients may improve the tired or sad look as well as decrease the upper eyelid hooding.

## 5.3.4 Patient Selection

Patients should be analyzed both in the static and dynamic positions. In the static analysis, the patients that will benefit from eyebrow lifting with botulinum toxin are those with a weak frontalis and strong depressors. Independent of age, the eyebrow has a low position; especially its lateral aspect, and fullness in the upper eyelid can also be observed. There may be static lines, depend-

**Table 5.3.** Muscles responsible for eyebrow positioning

| Muscle | Action | Synergists | Antagonists |
|--------|--------|------------|-------------|
| M. frontalis | Elevates the eyebrow and nasal skin | M. occipitalis | M. procerus, m. corrugator supercilii and m. orbicularis oculi |
| M. corrugator supercilii | Draws eyebrows medially and down | M. orbicularis oculi and m. procerus | M. frontalis |
| M. procerus | Depresses the medial end of the eyebrow | M. corrugator supercilii and m. orbicularis oculi | M. frontalis |
| M. orbicularis oculi | Orbital part: protrusion of the eyebrows and voluntary eyelid closure Palpebral part: closes lids during blinking Lacrimal part: draws lids and lacrimal papillae medially, compresses the lacrimal sac | M. corrugator supercilii and m. procerus | M. levator palpebrae superioris: for closing the eyelids; m. frontalis: protrusion of the eyebrows |

ing on the muscular behavior and age. In addition, the size of the forehead has to be considered since larger areas need more injection points and consequently higher doses.

The dynamic analysis should be done while talking to the patient in order to categorize them as kinetic, hyperkinetic or hypertonic. Kinetic patients only produce important eyebrow elevation if they want to denote surprise. Horizontal lines on the forehead are not visible when motionless. Hyperkinetic patients present eyebrow elevation independently of expressing surprise. Horizontal lines on the forehead due to frontalis over-contraction can be easily seen and disappear easily when motionless. Hypertonic patients can relax neither the eyebrow elevator nor the depressors. Lines are seen in both static and dynamic situations.

Kinetic patients are those that may present the best result: complete static and dynamic line removal and a nice elevation of the whole eyebrow.

A hyperkinetic m. frontalis may result in the Mephisto look due to the blocking of its medial fibers when treating the forehead. The Mephisto look may result from the over-contraction of the lateral frontalis fibers and absence of contraction of the medial fibers. It forms an undesired wrinkling just above the lateral part of the eyebrow. Hypertonic patients are difficult to treat; here treatment of the lateral brow might result in brow ptosis.

### 5.3.5 Technique

#### 5.3.5.1 Technique 1

BNT-A injections are placed into the upper lateral fibers of the m. orbicularis oculi pars orbitalis. One injection point approximately 0.5 cm above the orbital rim should be sufficient to target the lateral part of the m. orbicularis oculi. (Fig. 5.24)

#### 5.3.5.2 Technique 2

Another approach which is very efficient for lateral eyebrow lifting is the full blocking of the depressors and partial blocking of the medial fibers of the m. frontalis. The proper technique is described in the forehead and glabella sections (see Sects. 5.1 and 5.2; Fig. 5.25)

#### 5.3.5.3 Technique 3

A third method that can be used by more experienced injectors is the use of multiple injection points within the hair of the eyebrow. The injections should be superficial, with the needle pointing upwards. For lateral lifting only, three points are injected laterally to the supra-orbital foramen at the hemipupillary line (Fig. 5.26). If medial and lateral eyebrow lifting is desired, BNT should be distributed in five injection sites within the whole eyebrow. (Fig. 5.27)

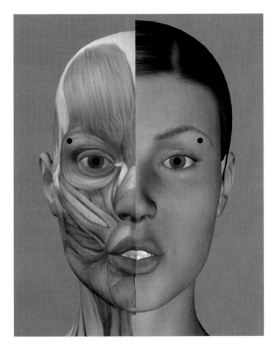

**Fig. 5.24.** Injection points for brow lift (technique 1). One point targeting the pars orbitalis of the m. orbicularis oculi for each side

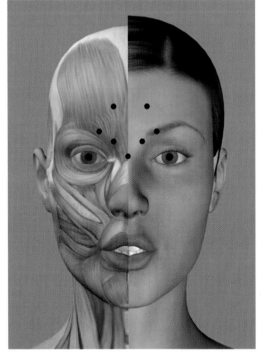

**Fig. 5.25.** Injection points for brow lift (technique 2). Here the central forehead region is treated

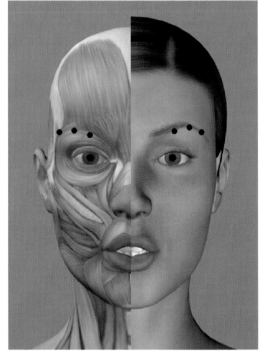

**Fig. 5.26.** Injection points for brow lift (technique 3). Here the lateral brow is treated with three injection points

Lateral Brow Lift

Technique 1

• One injection point approximately 0.5 cm above the orbital rim (Figs. 5.24 and 5.28)
  - Botox: 3–4 U per point
  - Dysport: 10–12 U per point

Technique 2

• Seven injection points (see Fig. 5.25)
  - Botox: mm. corrugatores: 3–5 U per point, m. procerus: 3–5 U, medial m. frontalis fibers : 2–6 U (two points)
  - Dysport: mm. corrugatores: 10–15 U per point, m. procerus: 10–15 U, medial m. frontalis fibers 6–15 U (two points)

Technique 3

  - Three to five injection points approximately 0.5 cm above the orbital rim (Figs. 5.26–5.33)

  - Botox: 1 U per point
  - Dysport: 3 U per point

The results may vary from patient to patient and the purpose of eyebrow lifting should always be taken into consideration. Technique 1 is suitable for mild lateral eyebrow lifting when the opponent elevating lateral fibers of the m. frontalis are strong enough to promote the lifting effect with the antagonist blocking (Fig. 5.34a,b). Technique 2 presents a good performance when only the lateral aspect of the eyebrow needs elevation and there are not many horizontal fibers in the forehead, only in the midline (Fig. 5.35a,b). Technique 3 is undoubtedly the most appropriate for medial, intermediate and lateral eyebrow lifting, but must be conducted only by experienced injectors (Fig. 5.36a,b).

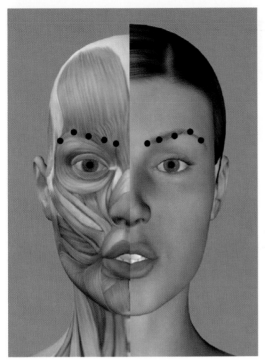

**Fig. 5.27.** Injection points for brow lift (technique 3). Here the total brow is treated with five injection points

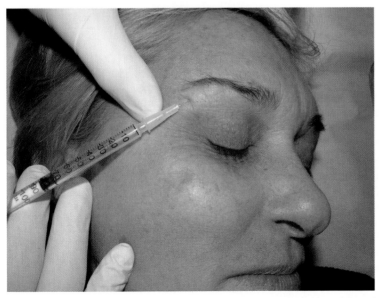

**Fig. 5.28.** This single injection point is useful for blocking the depressor effect of the upper lateral fibers of the m. orbicularis oculi pars orbitalis (technique 1). Care should be taken not to affect the laccrimal gland pump mechanism

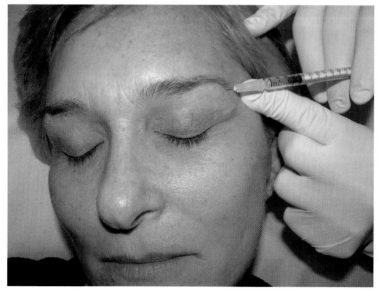

**Fig. 5.29.** Technique 3: first site: at this level, the injection should be superficial and within the eyebrow hair. It will block the blending fibers of the m. orbicularis oculi (upper lateral fibers) and m. frontalis (lower lateral fibers)

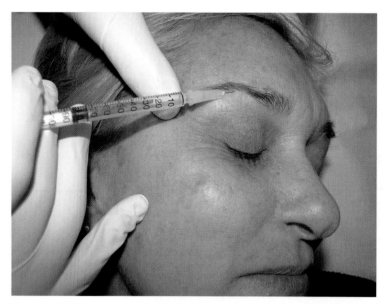

**Fig. 5.30.** Technique 3: second site: the injection is within the eyebrow hair, and superficial. The same blending fibers are blocked as mentioned in Fig. 5.29

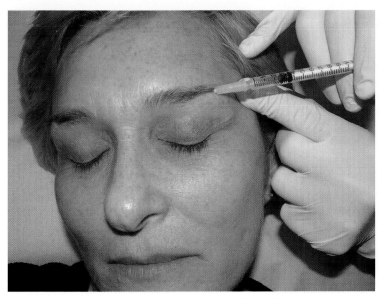

**Fig. 5.31.** Technique 3: third injection site: this can be the last point to promote lateral eyebrow lifting. The needle is inserted parallel to the skin into the direction of the supra-orbital foramen at the hemipupillary line

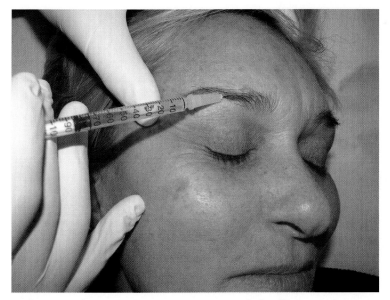

**Fig. 5.32.** Technique 3: the fourth injection site is used when the intermediate aspect of the eyebrow needs elevation. The needle is also inserted parallel to the skin and superficially. At this level, the fibers blocked include: m. frontalis lower fibers, m. corrugator inserting fibers, m. orbicularis oculi upper fibers

5

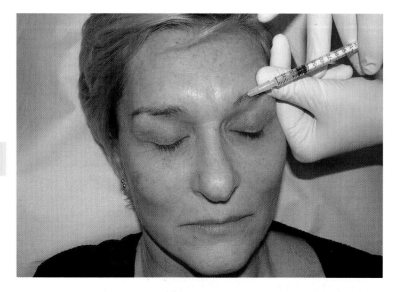

**Fig. 5.33.** Technique 3: the fifth point: at this level, the most medial aspect of the eyebrow is elevated. The same rule: needle parallel to the skin and superficial injection with low volume

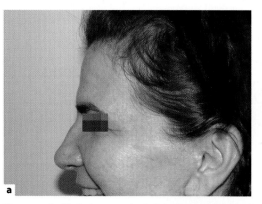 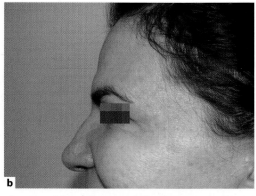

**Fig. 5.34a,b.** Technique 1: a single injection point at the lateral aspect of the eyebrow to inhibit the depressor effect of the upper lateral fibers of the m. orbicularis oculi

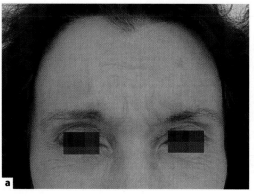 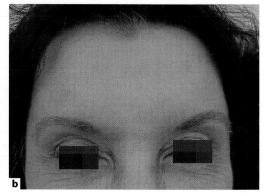

**Fig. 5.35a,b.** Technique 2: the blocking of the m.corrugator, m. procerus and only the medial fibers of the m. frontalis promotes eyebrow lifting

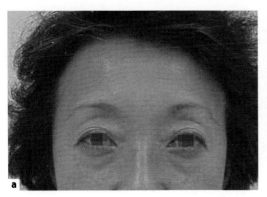 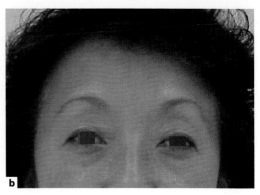

**Fig. 5.36a,b.** Technique 3 with five injection sites. Note that there is a lifting effect of the medial, intermediate and lateral aspects of the eyebrow. There is also improvement of the upper eyelid skin excess

## 5.3.6 Complications  !

Eyelid ptosis might rarely occur. In hypertonic patients BNT-A injections in the lateral part of the eyebrow might result in brow ptosis when excessive doses are used.

The technique of injection within the eyebrow (technique 3) may lead to upper eyelid ptosis if BNT-A is injected too deep and the needle directed downwards.

## 5.3.7 Tips and Tricks

■ Have the patient squeeze his eyes tight while you try to palpate the lateral parts of the m. orbicularis oculi. The injection point should be close to this area, but always above the orbital rim. Respect the learning curve: try technique 1 first, then technique 2 and after that technique 3 with three injection sites and with enough experience go to the five points.

## 5.3.8 References

Ahn MS et al. (2000) Temporal brow lift using botulinum toxin A. Plast Reconstr Surg 105(3):1129-35; discussion pp 1136-9

Balikian RV, Zimbler MS (2005) Primary and adjunctive uses of botulinum toxin type A in the periorbital region. Facial Plast Surg Clin North Am 13(4):583-90

Bulstrode NW, Grobbelaar AO (2002) Long-term prospective follow-up of botulinum toxin treatment for facial rhytides. Aesthetic Plast Surg 26(5):356-9

Chen AH, Frankel AS (2003) Altering brow contour with botulinum toxin. Facial Plast Surg Clin North Am 11(4):457-64

Cook BE Jr et al. (2001) Depressor supercilii muscle: anatomy, histology, and cosmetic implications. Ophthal Plast Reconstr Surg 17(6):404-11

de Almeida AR, Cernea SS (2001) Regarding browlift with botulinum toxin. Dermatol Surg 27(9):848

Frankel AS, Kamer FM (1998) Chemical browlift. Arch Otolaryngol Head Neck Surg 124(3):321-3

Huilgol SC et al. (1999) Raising eyebrows with botulinum toxin. Dermatol Surg 25(5):373-5; discussion p 376

Klein AW (2004) Botox for the eyes and eyebrows. Dermatol Clin 22(2):145-9

Koch RJ et al. (1997) Contemporary management of the aging brow and forehead. Laryngoscope 107(6):710-5

Kokoska MS et al. (2002) Modifications of eyebrow position with botulinum exotoxin A. Arch Facial Plast Surg 4(4):244-7

Kokoska MS et al. (2002) Modifications of eyebrow position with botulinum exotoxin A. Arch Facial Plast Surg 4(4):244-7

Le Louarn C (1998) Botulinum toxin and facial wrinkles: a new injection procedure. Ann Chir Plast Esthet 43(5):526-33

Le Louarn C (2001) Botulinum toxin A and facial lines: the variable concentration. Aesthetic Plast Surg 25(2):73-84

Le Louarn C (2004) Functional facial analysis after botulin on toxin injection. Ann Chir Plast Esthet 49(5):527-36

Lee CJ et al. (2006) The results of periorbital rejuvenation with botulinum toxin A using two different protocols. Aesthetic Plast Surg 30(1):65-70

Matarasso A, Hutchinson O (2003) Evaluating rejuvenation of the forehead and brow: an algorithm for selecting the appropriate technique. Plast Reconstr Surg 112(5):1467-9

Michelow BJ, Guyuron B (1997) Rejuvenation of the upper face. A logical gamut of surgical options. Clin Plast Surg 24(2):199-212

Muhlbauer W, Holm C (1998) Eyebrow asymmetry: ways of correction. Aesthetic Plast Surg 22(5):366-71

Ozsoy Z et al. (2005) A new technique applying botulinum toxin in narrow and wide foreheads. Aesthetic Plast Surg 29(5):368-72

Redaelli A, Forte R (2003) How to avoid brow ptosis after forehead treatment with botulinum toxin. J Cosmet Laser Ther 5(3-4):220-2

Sadick NS (2004) The cosmetic use of botulinum toxin type B in the upper face. Clin Dermatol 22(1):29-33

## 5.4  Crow's Feet and Lower Eyelid

*Mauricio de Maio*

### 5.4.1  Introduction

The eyes are among the most important areas of the face. Through the eyes, we communicate; we can understand each other's feelings.

The aging process in the eye area may lead to skin excess, eye bags, static and dynamic wrinkles and pigmentation disturbances. The wrinkling is usually only noticed during the smile and localized at the lateral part of the lower eyelid. It can simply appear as a fine skin creeping or be as deep as creases. In some cases, it can be seen without animation and is denominated as static wrinkles. Static wrinkles result from skin photo-damage and may be present in young people. They are usually worsened with animation and even more with skin excess.

Static and dynamic wrinkles have different etiology; however, they have a synergistic effect at the eye area. The presence of one component worsens the other and the single treatment of only one component does not promote an overall aesthetic improvement at the eye area. For example, if the patient presents skin excess, eye bags, scleral show, static and dynamic wrinkles and pigmented spots, the use of botulinum toxin will not produce the amazing outcome it usually does. Patients can become frustrated and may tend to see only the negative aspects of this treatment.

### 5.4.2  Anatomy

The m. orbicularis oculi is innervated by the temporal and zygomatic branches of the facial nerve. The m. orbicularis oculi arises from the nasal portion of the frontal bone, the frontal process of the maxilla, and the medial palpebral ligament.

It is composed of three portions: orbital, palpebral and lacrimal. The orbital portion forms the majority of the muscle bulk. Fibers are arranged in an elliptical pattern and present no interruption laterally. The superior orbital portion of the orbicularis oculi runs more superficially than the m. corrugator and blends medially into the frontalis. Laterally, the muscle extends over the temporal fascia. Inferiorly, it continues and covers the upper portion of the m. masseter. More medially, at the inferior orbital margin, its extensions cover the elevators of the upper lip.

The palpebral portion originates from the medial palpebral ligament and adjacent bone. It is subdivided into preseptal and pretarsal portions. The pretarsal fibers spread across the eyelids, the preseptal fibers course in front of the orbital septum and both fibers interdigitate laterally with the lateral palpebral raphe. The ciliary bundle is a small group of fine fibers lying at the palpebral margin.

The lacrimal portion has both superficial and deep heads that arise from the medial palpebral ligament and the posterior lacrimal crest. The fibers extend laterally to attach to the tarsi and to the lateral palpebral raphe (Table 5.4).

With normal muscle function, maximal orbital closure depends on the concentrated effort of all three portions of the m. orbicularis oculi. The contraction draws the skin and eyelids medially toward the bony attachments, which leads the lacrimal flow from the laterally and superiorly placed lacrimal gland toward the inferiorly and medially placed lacrimal sac. The orbital portion of the muscle is under voluntary control. The palpebral portion is under both voluntary and reflex control.

## 5.4.3  Aim of Treatment

The aim of treatment at the eye level includes reduction of hyperkinetic lines during animation and softening of hypertonic lines at rest.

## 5.4.4  Patient Selection

## 5.4.4.1  Crow's Feet

In general, patients with fair skin and blond or red hair show the effects of aging at an earlier stage. Blue or green eyes are more sensitive to daylight and as a consequence, squinting in bright sunlight may mechanically contribute to the lateral periorbital skin wrinkles. Patients with darker complexions have more protection, especially if their skin is more sebaceous. Eyelid skin wrinkling may also result from ultraviolet

**Table 5.4.** Characteristics of the m. orbicularis oculi

| Muscle | Action | Synergists | Antagonists |
|---|---|---|---|
| M. orbicularis oculi | Orbital part: protrusion of the eyebrows and voluntary eyelid closure. Palpebral part: closes lids during blinking. Lacrimal part: draws lids and lacrimal papillae medially, compresses the lacrimal sac | M. corrugator supercilii and m. procerus | M. levator palpebrae superioris: for closing the eyelids. M. occipitofrontalis: protrusion of the eyebrows |

ray damage, the desiccating effect of wind and from smoking.

Patients with thinner skin present very delicate wrinkling and patients with thicker skin present more prominent and deeper wrinkles. The more atrophic the skin is, the greater the quantity of fine wrinkles that may be found. Wrinkle extension also varies according to the muscle size, and some wrinkles can go down to the cheek area.

Eyebrow ptosis may contribute to upper eyelid skin excess and skin wrinkling. The lower eyelid may present with eye bags. Eye bags may result from the laxity of the orbicularis oculi and are considered to be a pseudo-herniation. It is not advisable to inject botulinum toxin for the treatment of crow's feet in patients with prominent eye-bags. If the muscle gets more relaxed, the eye-bags may get worse and a more tired look may result.

### 5.4.4.2 Lower Eyelid

When analyzing the lower eyelid, the quality of skin, presence of eye bags and wrinkling should be evaluated. The skin wrinkling in the lower eyelid results from the hyperkinetic behavior of the palpebral portion of the orbicularis oculi. The pretarsal portion of the muscle may produce orbicularis hypertrophy which reduces the palpebral aperture, especially in Asiatic patients. This periocular fold is known as 'jelly rolls'. The injection of botulinum toxin softens the bulginess at this site and promotes eye widening. It is a very nice treatment for Asiatic patients.

### 5.4.4.3 Eye Bags

Older patients present thinner and less elastic skin. The orbital septum is also less effective and weak. With this weakening, the inferior periorbital fat bulges and creates the suborbital eye bags

which results in a very tired appearance. Injection of botulinum toxin in patients with eye bags and scleral show is not advisable because they may get worse, so it should not be performed by inexperienced practitioners.

### 5.4.5 Technique

Good lighting avoids unwanted injection into blood vessels which may lead to bruising and ecchymosis.

After cleansing, marking is initiated. The patient should be asked to contract the eyes. The lateral extension of the crow's feet, and the presence of excessive wrinkling on the lower eyelid and nasal skin should be evaluated. Marking is undertaken according to the areas to be treated. Normal sized lateral extension needs only one row of three or four points; with longer lateral extensions, a second row is more laterally marked (Figs. 5.37–5.40).

The injector may position himself on the same side to be injected or on the opposite side. If the injector is positioned opposite to the patient, the needle will be pointed laterally and away from the patient's eye (Figs. 5.41 and 5.42).

Before the injection, stretching of the skin will be helpful to avoid perforating blood vessels. As the periorbital skin is thin, the needle may be inserted almost parallel to the skin and the botulinum toxin will diffuse to the underlying muscle. With deeper injection, it is more likely to produce skin bruising.

Injecting into the periorbital area is also useful for lifting the lateral aspect of the eyebrow. An upper lateral canthal injection blocks the depressor effect of the lateral fibers of the m. orbicularis oculi, which in conjunction with glabellar and the medial frontalis fibers may promote a lateral eyebrow lift (see Sect. 5.3 Brow lift).

The best injection site in the lower eyelid is at the pretarsal in the midpupilary line (Figs. 5.43–5.45). As well as the possibility of improving lower

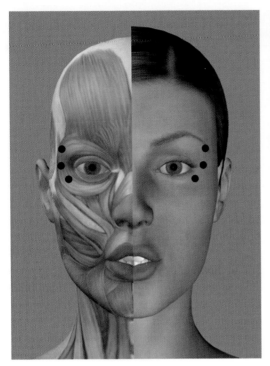

**Fig. 5.37.** Crow's feet: basic injection sites

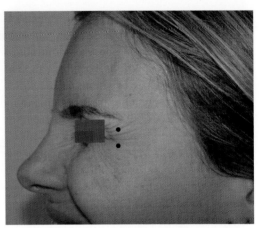

**Fig. 5.38.** Crow's feet: normal-sized lateral orbital fibers. The treatment of these patients is usually very satisfactory. The dynamic lines are basically limited to the orbital bone's lateral margin. Two points may be enough for such cases

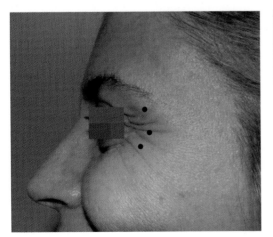

**Fig. 5.39.** Crow's feet: moderate-sized lateral orbital fibers: these are the typical patients for whom the conventional three points are indicated. The satisfaction rate is always high with correct technique

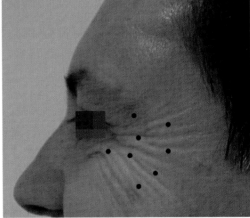

**Fig. 5.40.** Crow's feet with an excessive lateral orbital fibers extension: patients with this pattern of fibers should be treated in a different way. A greater number of sites should be injected, not necessarily increasing the final total dose too much. The microinjection technique is recommended here to reduce the risk of complications and to produce a better final result

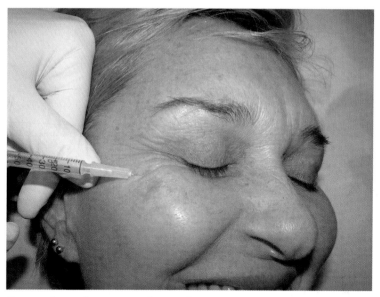

**Fig. 5.41.** Same side injection technique: the injector may be positioned on the same side as the wrinkles to be treated. Superficial injections are recommended to avoid bruising, since normally the vessels are deeper

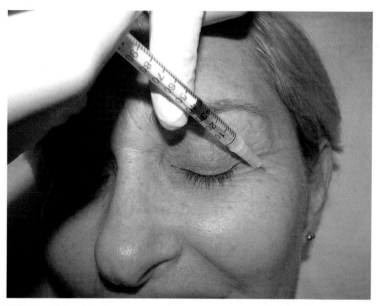

**Fig. 5.42.** Opposite side injection technique: if the injector is positioned on the opposite side to the crow's feet, the needle is directed outwards and there will be no danger for the eyeball

eyelid wrinkling, it produces a widening of the eye which leads to aesthetic enhancement. The needle should be inserted parallel to the skin so that a very superficial papule is seen. Any medial or lateral injection to the midpupillary line must be avoided or undertaken by very experienced injectors; otherwise complications may result.

Treatment of crow's feet and lower eyelid
- Three to five injection points
  - For crow's feet: three points lateral approximately 1 cm from the orbital rim
  - For lower eyelid: one to two injection points, infraorbital
- Injection technique: microinjection technique for the infraorbital points recommended
- Botox dose:
  - For crow's feet: total dose 6–15 U
  - For lower eyelid: total dose 1–2 U

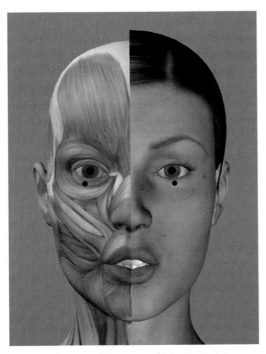

**Fig. 5.43.** Lower eyelid: pre-septal injection points

- Dysport dose:
  - For crow's feet: total dose 15–30 U
  - For lower eyelid: total dose 2–4 U

### 5.4.6 Results

Men usually accept a partial result and are satisfied with partial wrinkling reduction (Fig. 5.46a,b). Women are more demanding and require a more effective reduction in wrinkling.

In mild and moderate cases, periorbital wrinkling disappears in static and dynamic analysis (Figs. 5.47a,b–5.49a,b). In patients with photodamage, the result may be disappointing if they were not advised that combined therapy should be undertaken.

### 5.4.7 Complications

Ecchymosis and bruising may result from injection into the lower eyelid or deeper injections at the crow's feet. To prevent ecchymosis, the use of ice bags before and after injection may be helpful. Bruising may last from 7 to 15 days.

Analyzing the function of the three portions of the orbicularis oculi may lead to understanding of complications with its treatment. Injecting into the lateral fibers of the orbicularis oris should decrease the crow's feet. Complications such as upper lip asymmetry and cheek ptosis may result from injecting into the lowest extensions of the crow's feet at the m. zygomaticus major. Usually, these complications result from deep injections (see Fig. 7.1 and 7.2 in Sect. 7). At this level, the injection should be intradermal and of low volume. With excessive blocking of the palpebral portion, the lacrimal pump mechanism, forced eyelid closure and the blink reflex may be impaired. This may lead to dry eyes and corneal exposure, especially in older patients. To prevent lagophtalmos and scleral show, a snap test should be undertaken. If a sluggish reaction

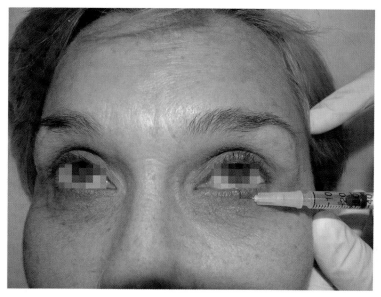

**Fig. 5.44.** Injection technique: pretarsal treatment with BNT-A should be undertaken with caution. The injection should be superficial, and papule formation should be the end-point

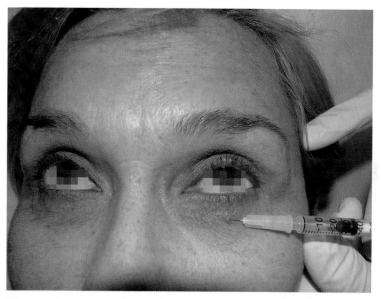

**Fig. 5.45.** The treatment of lower lid skin wrinkling may be conducted with BNT-A. Prominent eye bags, scleral show and a negative snap test should contra-indicate the injection at this level

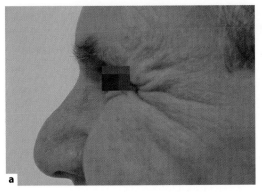
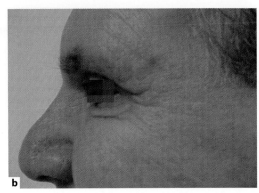

**Fig. 5.46a,b.** BNT-A treatment in men should be even more natural than in women. In general, men accept partial results very well and refuse excessive blocking

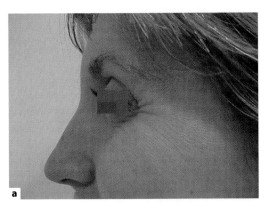
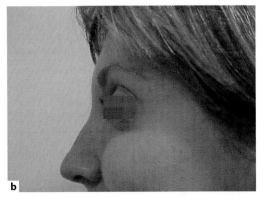

**Fig. 5.47a,b.** Before and after of a patient with normal-sized crow's feet. There is absolute removal of dynamic wrinkles

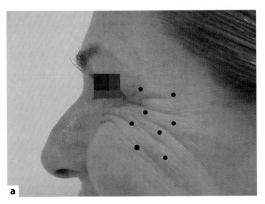
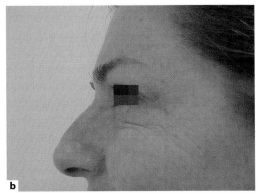

**Fig. 5.48a,b.** Before and after of a patient with a large lateral extension of crow's feet. To obtain a reduction of such wrinkling, multiple microinjections are recommended. The total dose should be evenly distributed among all points. Care should be taken with the lowest points; here microinjections at the zygoma level are mandatory

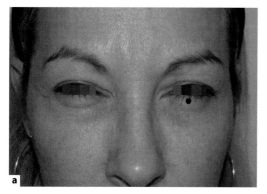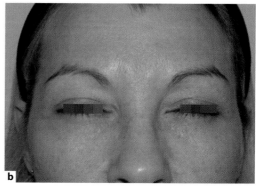

**Fig. 5.49a,b.** Hypertrophy of the m. orbicularis oculi pars palpebralis at the pre-tarsal area at the lower eyelid. After the injection of BNT-A, even with more squinting, there is no prominent contraction at this level. Note that although only the left eye has the injection site marked with a black dot, both sides were injected

results, any pretarsal injection in the lower eyelid should be avoided.

Pretarsal injections with the intention of decreasing lower eyelid wrinkling should be in the midpupillary line. Lateral injections to this point may lead to eyelid ectropion and rounded lateral canthus. Medial injections to the midpupillary line may cause epiphora and dry eyes.

Care must be taken while treating the lower eyelid. Blocking of the palpebral portion of the orbicularis oculi may lead to impairment of eye closure, for both voluntary and involuntary functions. If patients with eye bags are excessively treated, a worsening in eye bags may result. This is the so-called pseudo-herniation (Fig. 5.50a,b) and may be due to muscular weakness or lymphatic drainage impairment or both. There is no effective treatment for this. Lymphatic massages may promote a mild improvement. However, it is only the decrease of muscular blocking that will lead to an improvement. It is very important to have taken pictures of the patients before treatment. Some of them may believe and insist that the eye bags got worse after the treatment.

## 5.4.8  Tips and Tricks

- Avoid treating patients with prominent eye bags and skin excess; surgery is still the best option there (Fig. 5.51a,b). Prolonged wrinkling to the cheek area should be treated with intradermal injection and very low doses.

## 5.4.9  References

Batniji RK, Falk AN (2004) Update on botulinum toxin use in facial plastic and head and neck surgery. Curr Opin Otolaryngol Head Neck Surg 12(4):317-22

Baumann L et al. (2003) A double-blinded, randomized, placebo-controlled pilot study of the safety and efficacy of Myobloc (botulinum toxin type B)-purified neurotoxin complex for the treatment of crow's feet: a double-blinded, placebo-controlled trial. Dermatol Surg 29(5):508-15

Carruthers J et al. (2004) Consensus recommendations on the use of botulinum toxin type a in facial aesthetics. Plast Reconstr Surg 114(6 Suppl):1S-22S

Fagien S (2000) Intraoperative injection of botulinum toxin A into orbicularis oculi muscle for the treatment of crow's feet. Plast Reconstr Surg 105(6):2226-8

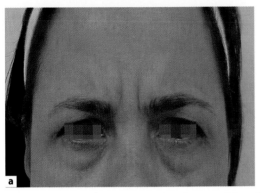 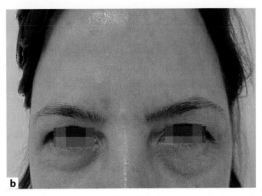

**Fig. 5.50a,b.** Note the worsening of the lower eyelid eye bags after the treatment of the glabella and crow's feet with BNT-A

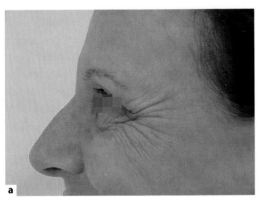 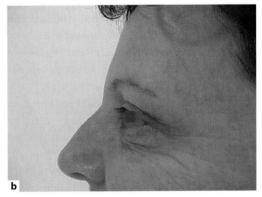

**Fig. 5.51a,b.** The treatment of the crow's feet may accentuate lower skin excess. Either lower skin removal with surgery or lower eyelid injection with BNT-A should be undertaken to avoid undesirable results

Flynn TC et al. (2003) Botulinum A toxin (BOTOX) in the lower eyelid: dose-finding study. Dermatol Surg 29(9):943-50; discussion 950-1

Guerrissi JO (2000) Intraoperative injection of botulinum toxin A into orbicularis oculi muscle for the treatment of crow's feet. Plast Reconstr Surg 104(6):2219-25

Kane MA (2003) Classification of crow's feet patterns among caucasian women: the key to individualizing treatment. Plast Reconstr Surg 112(5 Suppl):33S-39S

Klein AW (2004) Botox for the eyes and eyebrows. Dermatol Clin 22(2):145-9

Klein AW (2004) Contraindications and complications with the use of botulinum toxin. Clin Dermatol 22(1):66-75

Guerrissi JO (2003) Intraoperative injection of botulinum toxin A into the orbicularis oculi muscle for the treatment of crow's feet. Plast Reconstr Surg 112(5 Suppl):161S-3S

Lee CJ et al. (2006) The results of periorbital rejuvenation with botulinum toxin A using two different protocols. Aesthetic Plast Surg 30(1):65-70

Levy JL et al. (2004) Botulinum toxin A: a 9-month clinical and 3D in vivo profilometric crow's feet wrinkle formation study. J Cosmet Laser Ther 6(1):16-20

Lowe NJ et al. (2005) Double-blind, randomized, placebo-controlled, dose-response study of the safety and efficacy of botulinum toxin type A in subjects with crow's feet. Dermatol Surg 31(3):257-62

Lowe NJ et al. (2002) Bilateral, double-blind, randomized comparison of 3 doses of botulinum toxin type A and placebo in patients with crow's feet. J Am Acad Dermatol 47(6):834-40

Matarasso SL, Matarasso A (2001) Treatment guidelines for botulinum toxin type A for the periocular region and a report on partial upper lip ptosis following injections to the lateral canthal rhytids. Plast Reconstr Surg 108(1):208-14; discussion pp 215-7

Naik MN et al. (2005) Botulinum toxin in ophthalmic plastic surgery. Indian J Ophthalmol 53(4):279-88

Semchyshyn N, Sengelmann RD (2003) Botulinum toxin A treatment of perioral rhytides. Dermatol Surg 29(5):490-5; discussion p 495

Flynn TC et al. (2003) Botulinum A toxin (BOTOX) in the lower eyelid: dose-finding study. Dermatol Surg 29(9):943-50; discussion pp 950-1

Flynn TC et al. (2001) Botulinum-A toxin treatment of the lower eyelid improves infraorbital rhytides and widens the eye. Dermatol Surg 27(8):703-8

Balikian RV, Zimbler MS (2005) Primary and adjunctive uses of botulinum toxin type A in the periorbital region. Facial Plast Surg Clin North Am 13(4):583-90

Frankel AS (1999) Botox for rejuvenation of the periorbital region. Facial Plast Surg 15(3):255-62

Kim DW et al. (2003) Botulinum toxin A for the treatment of lateral periorbital rhytids. Facial Plast Surg Clin North Am 11(4):445-51

Lee CJ et al. (2006) The results of periorbital rejuvenation with botulinum toxin A using two different protocols. Aesthetic Plast Surg 30(1):65-70

Spiegel JH (2005) Treatment of periorbital rhytids with botulinum toxin type A: maximizing safety and results. Arch Facial Plast Surg 7(3):198-202

may be naturally present in some patients when they smile, laugh, frown or speak. However, they may appear or worsen after treatment with BNT-A, especially in the crow's feet and glabella area, leading to the so-called BNT-sign. Patients usually blame the injector if those lines result from the injection of BNT-A for any cosmetic purpose.

When blocking a specific muscle, it is very likely that its synergistic muscle may contract as well and sometimes may even react with over-contraction. When the eye and nose complex is under animation, there is parallel contraction of the mm. corrugatores, m. procerus, m. nasalis and mm. orbiculares oculi and, depending on the patient, the upper lip elevators as well.

The most common treatment with botulinum toxin in the upper third includes the blocking of the m. frontalis, mm. corrugatores, m. procerus and m. orbicularis oculi. If the m. nasalis is not treated, undesired bunny lines may result. Depending on the skin complexion, there will be more or less wrinkle formation. For example, patients with thin skin and fair complexion are more prone to develop wrinkling on the nasal dorsum and lateral walls. Sometimes, there are wrinkling extensions to the lower eyelid. Darker complexion and oily skin produce thick wrinkling and are usually limited to the nasal dorsum.

The choice of treating the bunny lines concomitant with crow's feet or glabella area will depend on the patient. If they are not treated during the same session, and become too evident after the treatment, they can be treated afterwards.

## 5.5  Bunny Lines

### Mauricio de Maio

### 5.5.1  Introduction

Bunny lines are defined as those wrinkling on the lateral and/or dorsal aspect of the nose. They

## 5.5.2  Anatomy

The skin is thinner and more mobile in the upper two thirds of the nose, and it is thicker and more adherent in the lower third. The thinner and older the skin is, the more wrinkling is to be formed on the nasal dorsum.

The nose contains three main muscles: the m. procerus, the m. nasalis and the m. depressor septi nasi. The m. procerus draws the medial part of the eyebrow down. It originates at the nasal root and blends with the frontalis fibers. The m. depressor septi nasi drops the tip of the nose when contracted. Finally, the m. nasalis is the most important one for promoting the bunny lines and will be the main focus of this section. Although the m. levator labii superioris alaeque nasi is not an intrinsic nasal muscle, it may contribute to the bunny lines due to its medial fibers.

The m. nasalis originates in the transition from the nasal bone with the maxilla and inserts into the aponeurosis of the nasal dorsum. It looks like an upside-down horseshoe, with the upper or curved part formed by transverse fibers on the nasal dorsum. Its action is to narrow the nostrils (also denominated as m. compressor naris). The transverse fibers of the m. nasalis lead, when contracted, to the lateral nasal lines (bunny lines) and to additional lines in the internal infra-ocular region. The two lower parts of the m. nasalis run vertically down the sides of the nose (also known as the dilator nasi) and their action is to open the nostrils (Table 5.5).

## 5.5.3 Aim of the Treatment

The aim of the treatment is to reduce bunny lines; either those naturally present or those appearing after treatment of the glabella and crow's feet area with BNT.

## 5.5.4 Patient Selection

Bunny lines may be treated alone or in conjunction with the treatment of the crow's feet and glabellar lines. Kinetic patients usually do not present lines on the nasal dorsum when smiling and concomitant treatment with crow's feet may not be necessary.

In static analysis, hyperkinetic and hypertonic patients may present wrinkles on the nasal dorsum. The presence of those lines at rest indicates the need for bunny line treatment concomitant with crow's feet and glabellar lines.

During animation, patients should be asked to laugh, to sniff and to squint intensely as if a very bright light is before their eyes. Usually, bunny lines are not present in kinetic patients with a mild smile. They only become evident when smiling at maximum contraction. In hyperkinetic patients, bunny lines are found with a mild smile and worsen at maximum contraction. Due to constant squinting, the m. nasalis may become hypertrophic and may reduce the duration of effect of BNT-A at the nasal level.

Bunny lines may be limited to the nose, with extension to lower eyelid and reach the nasal

**Table 5.5.** Characteristics of the m. nasalis and the m. levator labii superioris alaeque nasi

| Muscle | Action | Synergists | Antagonists |
|---|---|---|---|
| M. nasalis | Compression naris: compresses the nasal aperture Dilator naris: widens the anterior nasal aperture | Medial parts of the m. levator labii superioris alaeque nasi and m. depressor septi | None |
| M. levator labii superioris alaeque nasi | Medial part: dilates the nostril Lateral part: raises and everts the upper lip | Medial part: m. dilator nasi Lateral part: m. levator labii superioris, m. zygomaticus major and minor and m. levator anguli oris | M. depressor anguli oris and m. orbicularis oris |

flare. Depending on the patient, they may be present only at the lateral aspect of the nasal dorsum or at the upper aspect of the nasal bone (Fig. 5.52a,b).

### 5.5.5 Technique

After static and dynamic evaluation, the injection points can be marked on the lateral and upper aspect of the nasal bone if needed. The injection should be very superficial because the skin at this level is very thin and contact with the periosteum may be painful (Fig. 5.53). The needle should be at an angle of 30°, because it is easier to avoid touching the periosteum. There is an evident papule or wheal formation after the injection. Care should be taken with blood vessels at this level, otherwise bruising may result.

A total dose of 2–5 U of Botox or 6–15 U Dysport should be distributed on both lateral sides (Fig. 5.54). In selected cases, extra doses from 1 to 2 U Botox or 3 to 5 U Dysport may be injected in the midline (Figs. 5.55 and 5.56). It is important not to inject too laterally down the nasal sidewalls; otherwise, the levator labii superioris alaeque nasi may be blocked and upper lip ptosis and asymmetry may result.

Care should be taken to avoid injection into the angular vessels which would produce bruising and ecchymosis. Partial or no effect often results from inadvertent injection into the blood vessels.

Patients usually get disappointed if bunny lines result after the blocking of the glabellar and forehead lines (Fig. 5.57a,b). As soon as evidenced, the patient should be treated. If, during the pre-treatment evaluation, bunny lines appear with frowning, concomitant treatment with the glabellar lines must be undertaken (Fig. 5.58a,b).

Treatment of bunny lines
- Two injection points, one for each side of the nose. In certain cases an additional medial point may be added
- Botox dose: 2–5 U total dose for the two points, 1–2 U for the extra point
- Dysport dose: 6–15 U total dose for the two points, 3–5 U for the extra point

### 5.5.6 Complications

The most common complication with the treatment of bunny lines is the presence of ecchymo-

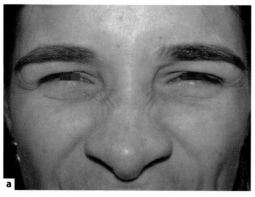
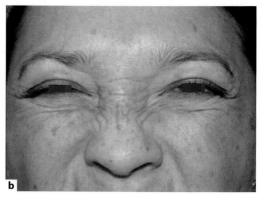

**Fig. 5.52a,b.** Note the difference between the two patterns of bunny lines. The patient in a has lines predominantly limited to the lateral aspect of the nose. The patient in b has bunny line extensions to the nasal dorsum, lower eyelid and nasal flare. It is easier to improve those lines in the first patient. The second patient presents a more complex situation

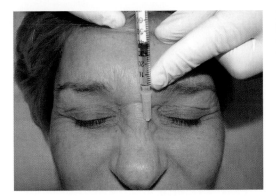

**Fig. 5.53.** The injection technique on the lateral bunny lines should be superficial and a wheal formation is desirable. Care should be taken not to inject into blood vessels to avoid bruising

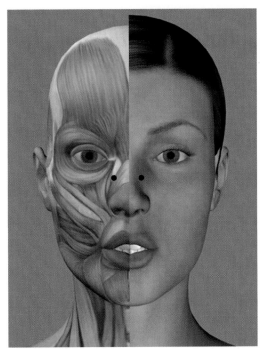

**Fig. 5.54.** Injection technique: lateral injection points

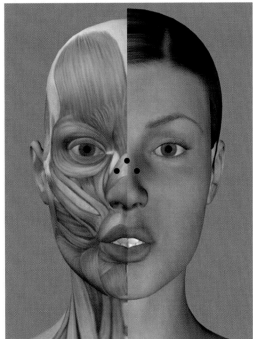

**Fig. 5.55.** Injection technique: lateral and dorsal injection points

5

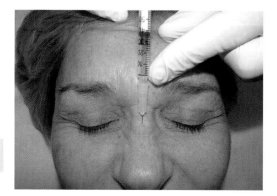

**Fig. 5.56.** Some patients may also present lines on the nasal dorsum. Injection should be superficial as well. Here bruising after the injection can be quite common

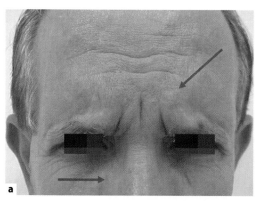

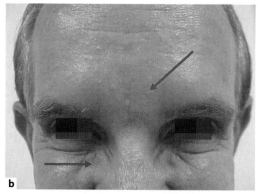

a                           b

**Fig. 5.57a,b.** This patient was submitted to BNT-A in the glabella, forehead and crow´s feet. Note that during animation, there is no contraction of the m. nasalis. After blocking the specific muscles, bunny lines appeared due to the blocking of upper third muscles of the face except the m. nasalis

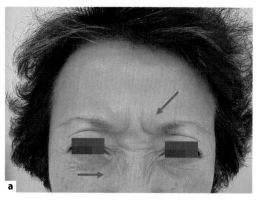

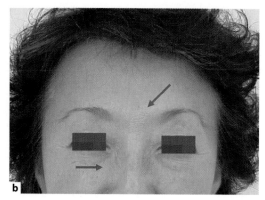

a                           b

**Fig. 5.58a,b.** This patient showed bunny lines while frowning, before treatment. In these patients it is recommended that the bunny lines are treated at the same time as the glabella. After injection with BNT-A an improvement in both glabellar and bunny lines can be observed

sis or hematoma. An unsatisfactory result may be due to inadvertent injection into blood vessels. Major problems such as diplopia and upper lip ptosis may result from inadvertent blocking of the rectus inferioris or medialis and the levator labii superioris alaeque nasi, respectively. More serious complications may include speaking and chewing difficulty.

### 5.5.7 Tips and Tricks

■ Bunny line treatment really does produce an upgrade in cosmetic evaluation in patients treated with BNT-A. So, do not forget them!

### 5.5.8 References

Ahn KY et al. (2000) Botulinum toxin A for the treatment of facial hyperkinetic wrinkle lines in Koreans. Plast Reconstr Surg 105(2):778-84

Carruthers J, Carruthers A (2003) Aesthetic botulinum A toxin in the mid and lower face and neck. Dermatol Surg 29(5):468-76

Carruthers J et al. (2004) Consensus recommendations on the use of botulinum toxin type A in facial aesthetics. Plast Reconstr Surg 114(6 Suppl):1S-22S

Huang W et al. (2000) Browlift with botulinum toxin. Dermatol Surg 26(1):55-60

## 5.6 Nose

*Maurício de Maio*

### 5.6.1 Introduction

The volume, mass and shape of the three aesthetic thirds and the magnitude of nasal promi-

nence and projection determine what we may consider as aesthetic beauty. Any diminution or enhancement in size in one facial zone directly and inversely impacts the others. The nose is such an important landmark in facial beauty that even slight modifications may lead to dramatic changes. The tip of the nose plays an important role in nasal beauty. Preferably, the nasolabial angle in women should be 95–100° and in men, approximately 90–95°.

Aging processes may alter the shape of the nose. It is primarily the drooping of the nasal tip and the increasing prominence of the dorsal hump which can be observed. There is a relative shortening of the lower third of the face and a relative lengthening of the nose which, together with a loss of support of the lateral cartilages, gives the appearance of a drooping tip and accentuates any dorsal convexity.

### 5.6.2 Anatomy

The nose contains three main muscles: the m. procerus, the m. nasalis and the m. depressor septi nasi. The m. procerus has two venters that originate at the nose root and the insertion fibers are intertwined with those of the frontal. Its action is more concentrated at the glabella area. It depresses the medial portion of the eyebrows and forms the horizontal line on the glabella. The m. nasalis originates in the transition from the nasal bone with the maxilla and inserts in the aponeurosis of the nasal dorsum. It moves the nose and is auxiliary to the opening of the nostrils. It forms the lateral lines on the nose.

The most important muscle that acts on the position of the nose tip is the m. depressor septi nasi. Its origin is at the base of the nasal septum and it blends with the fibers of the orbicularis oris. Its fibers are longitudinal and with contraction, it shortens the upper lip and can decrease tip projection on animation. There are three distinct variations of this muscle. The more common type I depressor septi muscles (62%) are visible and identifiable and present full interdigitation with the orbicularis oris from their origin at the medial crural footplate. Type II muscles (22%) are also identifiable but insert into the periosteum and present little or no interdigitation with the orbicularis oris. The least common type III muscles (16%) present no or only a rudimentary depressor septi muscle (Table 5.6).

### 5.6.3 Aim of Treatment

The purpose of blocking the depressor septi nasi with BNT-A is to elevate the tip of the nose at rest and avoid its drooping during a smile.

The blocking of the dilator nasi may decrease the nostril aperture in certain cases.

### 5.6.4 Patient Selection

Routine pre-treatment examination should easily identify those young patients who present a drooping nasal tip and upper lip shortening when smiling. The shape of the face is usually convex with a prominent nose and an underdeveloped chin. Those patients are mainly mouth breathers.

Another situation that may be found with the drooping tip is during the aging process. With nose elongation and muscle changes, the tip of the nose tends to drop mainly in those patients with acute nasolabial angles.

In frontal view, there is an evident downward movement when the patient smiles, especially at maximum contraction. On profile analysis, the nasolabial angle is usually less than 90° at rest and decreases when the patient smiles.

Excessive opening of the nasal flare may be found in some individuals during physical or emotional stress. The dilator nasi contraction may cause this excessive opening.

### 5.6.5 Technique

The patient should be evaluated according to the length of the upper lip and the nasal-labial angle. There are two ways of blocking the m. depressor septi nasi with BNT-A: through the skin and intra-orally. As the nasal area is quite sensitive, the use of topical anesthesia or ice bags to reduce the pain is advisable.

As mentioned above, there are three different anatomical patterns for the m. depressor septi nasi. That is one of the main reasons why the outcome may vary from patient to patient.

### 5.6.5.1 Technique 1

The trans-cutaneous approach is carried out by marking the injection points at the base of the

**Table 5.6.** Characteristics of the m. nasalis and the m. depressor septi

| Muscle | Action | Synergists | Antagonists |
|---|---|---|---|
| M. nasalis | Compression naris: compresses the nasal aperture Dilator naris: widens the anterior nasal aperture | Medial parts of the m. levator labii superioris alaeque nasi and m. depressor septi | None |
| M. depressor septi | Draws the nasal tip downwards and thereby constricts the nostrils | M. nasalis | M. dilator nasi |

columella at the medial crural footplate. Two points are marked, one at each side of the medial crura, and the injection is started (Fig. 5.59). As the fibers of the m. depressor septi nasi are intertwined with those of the m. orbicularis oris, the injection should be superficial. Usually, the first third of the 30-gauge needle is inserted (+/- 3–4 mm). The dose at each side is 1–2 U Botox or 4–6 U Dysport.

### 5.6.5.2 Technique 2

Another option for the trans-cutaneous approach is a single injection point at the columella base between the two medial crura (Fig. 5.60). At this level, the muscle is also superficial and 2–3 U Botox or 5–9 U Dysport can be injected (Figs. 5.61 and 5.62).

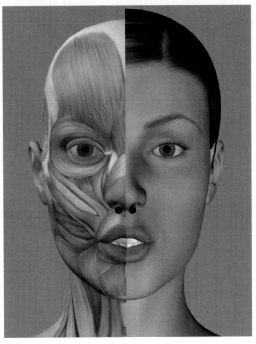

**Fig. 5.59.** Transcutaneous approach: two injection points, one at each side of the medial crura

### 5.6.5.3 Technique 3

The intra-oral approach is less painful but it may be considered more difficult by some to inject into the correct level. The same needle may be used; however, the injection must preferably be undertaken in two sites right beside the frenulum. The m. depressor septi nasi fibers are intertwined with the orbicularis oris, so at least half of the 30 gauge needle should be inserted with its bevel directed to the columella base. A total dose of 1–3 U Botox or 3–7 U Dysport at each side should be injected.

Treatment of the m. depressor septi nasi
Technique 1
- Two transcutaneous lateral injection points (Fig. 5.59)
- Botox dose: 1–2 U per side
- Dysport dose: 4–6 U per side

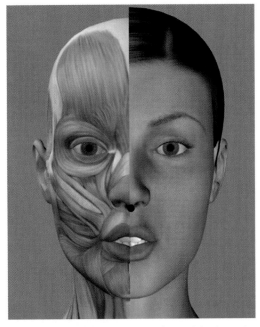

**Fig. 5.60.** Transcutaneous approach: one injection point at the base of the columella

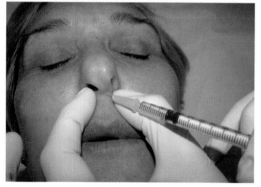

**Fig. 5.61.** Injection of BNT-A at the base of the collumella. The fibers of the m. depressor septi nasi run close to the medial crural footplate. This location is ideal for patients with normal or short upper lips

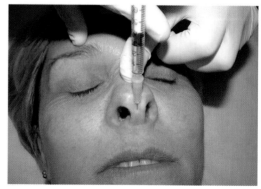

**Fig. 5.62.** The m. depressor septi nasi fibers run upwards to the tip of the nose. Injection of BNT-A at the middle portion of the collumella is ideal for those patients who present a long upper lip

Technique 2
- One transcutaneous medial injection point (Figs. 5.60– 5.62)
- Botox dose: 2–3 U
- Dysport dose: 5–9 U

Technique 3
- Two intraoral lateral injection points
- Botox dose: 1–3 U per side
- Dysport dose: 3–7 U per side

To inject into the dilator nasi, the patient should be asked to breathe in and the exact location of the muscle movement should be marked. The skin at this level is much adhered to the cartilage and injection may be quite painful. The bevel should be turned downwards, especially in patients with large pores in the skin. During the treatment, it is common to see an immediate bleaching with the injection, which subsides shortly after. A total of 1–2 U Botox and 3–5 U Dysport should be injected (Fig. 5.63a,b).

Treatment of the m. dilator nasi
- One injection point
- Botox dose: 1–2 U total dose
- Dysport dose: 3 -5 U total dose

## 5.6.6 Results

The injection of botulinum toxin in the m. depressor septi nasi may achieve the following goals: 1. Enhancement of the nasolabial angle in static and dynamic positions, 2. Slight upper lip lengthening, 3. Slight fullness of the upper lip, 4. Elevation of the tip of the nose, 5. Improvement of the horizontal lines between the upper lip rim and the nasal base (Figs. 5.64a,b and 5.65a,b).

## 5.6.7 Complications

Complications are rare when patients are selected properly and correct techniques are used. Complications such as hematoma and edema hardly ever happen. Pain is the adverse event most often reported. Injection into the dilator nasi barely results in complications. In contrast, at the nasal base, over-blocking of the m. depressor septi nasi may result in upper lip ptosis. This is more prone in patients with a long upper lip in whom any relaxation may lead to elongation at the medial tubercle and philtrum. As a result, the central upper incisors become hidden and through the contraction of the m. zygomaticus major with upper lateral pulling of the lips, the 'joker' smile may result.

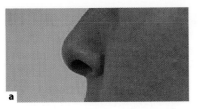 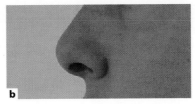

**Fig. 5.63a,b.** The blocking of the m. dilator nasi may reshape the nostril and decrease its size, leading to a more delicate appearance of the nose

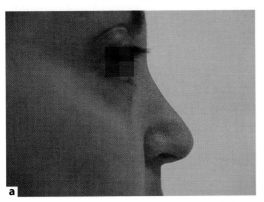 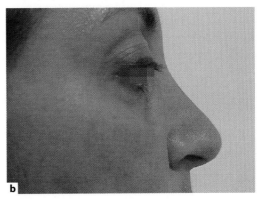

**Fig. 5.64a,b.** The contraction of the depressor of the septum makes the tip of the nose rounded and inclined downwards. The injection of BNT-A promotes elevation of the tip of the nose and a more gracious profile

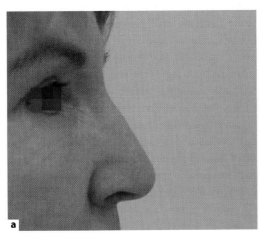 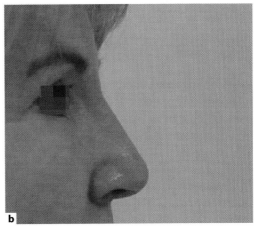

**Fig. 5.65a,b.** The blocking of the m. depressor septi nasi promotes a slight lifting and upward rotation of the tip of the nose. It gives a more youthful appearance

If the zygomaticus major traction is excessive and there is social impairment for the patient, a very careful injection at the upper part of the modiolus where the m. zygomaticus major inserts should be conducted. A next-to-nothing dose (0.5 U Botox ,1 U Dysport) must be carried out very superficially. Extra tiny doses may be injected at the same level with 7 days apart until the desired effect is obtained. To improve upper lip ptosis, very little can be done. In general, 15 days after the injection there is some recovery of the muscle tonus with upper lip lifting and aesthetic improvement.

### 5.6.8  Tips and Tricks

- The best candidates to start treatment of the m. depressor septi nasi are those with a short upper lip and preferably a gummy smile. Even if there is upper lip lengthening after the BNT-A injection, the patient will benefit cosmetically.

### 5.6.9  References

Rees TD (1978) Rhinoplasty in the older patient. Ann Plast Surg 1:27

Patterson C (1980) The aging nose: characteristics and correction. Otolaryngol Clin North Am 13:275

Rohrich RJ et al. (2000) Importance of the depressor septi nasi muscle in rhinoplasty: anatomic study and clinical application. Plast Reconstr Surg 105:376

Batniji RK, Falk AN (2004) Update on botulinum toxin use in facial plastic and head and neck surgery. Curr Opin Otolaryngol Head Neck Surg 12(4):317-22

Carruthers J et al. (2004) Consensus recommendations on the use of botulinum toxin type a in facial aesthetics. Plast Reconstr Surg 114(6 Suppl):1S-22S

Dayan SH, Kempiners JJ (2005) Treatment of the lower third of the nose and dynamic nasal tip ptosis with Botox. Plast Reconstr Surg 115(6):1784-5

De Maio M (2004) The minimal approach: an innovation in facial cosmetic procedures. Aesthetic Plast Surg 28(5):295-300

Kane MA (2003) The effect of botulinum toxin injections on the nasolabial fold. Plast Reconstr Surg 112(5 Suppl):66S-72S; discussion pp 73S-74S

Le Louarn C (2001) Botulinum toxin A and facial lines: the variable concentration. Aesthetic Plast Surg 25(2):73-84

Tamura BM et al. (2005) Treatment of nasal wrinkles with botulinum toxin. Dermatol Surg 31(3):271-5

## 5.7  Nasolabial Fold

### *Mauricio de Maio*

### 5.7.1  Introduction

One of the aging signs in the mid third of the face is the prominent nasolabial fold. Facial cosmetic surgeries are unable to solve this issue by muscle traction and skin removal alone. Usually, the best treatment for deep nasolabial folds is the injection of fillers. In some cases, though, the single use of fillers in the nasolabial fold may produce undesirable results, especially when the main component that produces the prominent nasolabial fold is muscular over-contraction. Cosmetic practitioners tend to inject excessive amounts of fillers to fill what should not be filled, but blocked. Overcorrection of the folds with fillers can result in a bizarre appearance, making patients look fat or swollen.

The natural muscle action on the nasolabial fold may express different emotions. When it is the upper part that is deepened, it expresses disgust or anger. In contrast, when it is the lower part, it means grief, sadness or joy.

Due to the quantity of muscles that act at the perioral area, the treatment of the nasolabial fold must be carried out with great care. The presence of mild asymmetries after treatment is not rare and should be promptly corrected when diagnosed. It is not easy to determine the proper dose the first time we treat a new patient. For this reason, it is advisable that the treatment be conducted in two steps until the correct dose is determined.

It should be emphasized that the presence of a natural nasolabial fold is not a negative cosmetic sign. It is its depth and prominence that may affect and disturb facial expression and beauty. Also, the complete elimination of it could be detrimental to facial harmony.

## 5.7.2 Anatomy

The nasolabial fold extends from the upper lateral part of the nasal flare down to the oral commissure. It can vary from individual to individual: be complete absent or flat or even very deep with skin excess and premaxillary deficiency. It can stop laterally to the oral commissure or go downward to the chin area. In general, a prominent nasolabial fold may result from more than one etiology. It can result from the loss of skin thickness over the sulcus; from the presence of redundant skin drooping over the sulcus; from excessive fat deposits laterally to the sulcus; from ptosis and/or laxity of the malar fat pad and from muscular hyperactivity. In older patients, more than one factor usually causes the prominent nasolabial fold.

With the aging of the face, there is a loss of subcutaneous fullness which is associated with youth. The fat loss results in a less tightened skin which produces folds and wrinkles. The nasolabial fold becomes more prominent and unintentional emotions are expressed. With the loss of biomechanical support, the skin suffers the action of muscular hyperactivity even more.

The muscles at the nasolabial level, from medially to laterally, are the m. levator labii superioris alaeque nasi, m. levator labii superioris, m. zygomaticus minor, m. zygomaticus major and at a deeper level, the m. levator anguli oris. It is important to emphasize that the zygomaticus major has little or no effect on the nasolabial fold.

The m. levator labii superioris is the main elevator of the upper lip and functions to create and move the middle portion of the nasolabial fold. It originates from the lower margin of the orbit, above the infraorbital foramen and below the orbicularis oculi. It continues downward between the levator labii superioris alaeque nasi and zygomaticus minor and inserts into the central and lateral aspects of the upper lip. It elevates and everts the upper lip.

Another important muscle that acts upon the nasolabial fold is the m. levator labii superioris alaeque nasi. It originates from the frontal process of the maxilla and descends and divides itself into two muscle bundles: the most medial smaller fibers insert into the nasal cartilage and the skin of the nose and a larger and more lateral bundle continues downward and inserts into the upper lip, merging its fibers with the m. levator labii superioris and with the m. orbicularis oris. The m. levator labii superioris alaeque nasi creates the medial most upper portion of the nasolabial fold. Its medial nasal muscle bundle dilates the nostril and displaces the sulcus laterally, elevating the nasolabial fold. The labial muscle bundles evert and elevate the upper lip (Table 5.7).

## 5.7.3 Aim of Treatment

The aim of the treatment of the nasolabial fold with botulinum toxin is to reduce muscular hyperactivity at this level. The blocking of the m. levator labii superioris or m. levator labii superioris alaeque nasi should flatten or smooth the prominent nasolabial fold.

## 5.7.4 Patient Selection

Deep or prominent nasolabial folds are considered signs of aging. Young people who have deep nasolabial folds consider themselves to be older than they really are. It is very important to examine the patient in static and dynamic positions.

**Table 5.7.** Characteristics of the m. levator labii superioris and the m. levator labii superioris alaeque nasi

| Muscle | Action | Synergists | Antagonists |
|---|---|---|---|
| M. levator labii superioris | Elevates and everts the upper lip. Creates and moves the middle portion of the nasolabial fold. | Lateral part of m. levator labii superioris alaeque nasi, m. levator anguli oris and mm. zygomaticus major and minor | M. depressor anguli oris and m. orbicularis oris |
| M. levator labii superioris alaeque nasi | Medial part: dilates the nostril Lateral part: raises and everts the upper lip Creates the most upper portion of the nasolabial fold. | Medial part: m. dilator nasi Lateral part: m. levator labii superioris, m. zygomaticus major and minor and m. levator anguli oris | M. depressor anguli oris and m. orbicularis oris |

In static analysis, there should be a prominent nasolabial fold. The surrounding structures such as cheeks, lips and chin should also be evaluated. If the prominent nasolabial fold is surrounded by atrophic tissues and the upper lateral part of the nasal flare is flat, it is likely that the best treatment should be the injection of fillers. In contrast, if the surrounding tissues are prominent and there is a bulging area at the upper lateral part of the nasal flare, the injection of botulinum toxin should be considered.

In the dynamic analysis, patients should be asked to smile at maximum contraction. The most upper part of the nasolabial fold should be even more pronounced. Palpation at this level confirms the contraction of the levator labii superioris alaeque nasi where it divides its fibers to the nasal flare and upper lip.

The ideal patients to start with the injection of BNT-A are those with a short distance between the vermillion border and the nasal base (short upper lip). When smiling, these patients should present excessive gum exposure. Patients with a long upper lip (vermillion border to nasal base) should be carefully treated, because one of the undesirable results of the injection at the nasolabial fold level is the upper lip lengthening.

### 5.7.5 Technique

After proper patient assessment, the bulging area at the upper part of the nasolabial fold is marked. Usually, no anesthetic is required. In more sensitive patients, topical anesthetic creams can be applied 20 minutes before the treatment. The injection should be superficial at an angle of 30° and only the first third (+/- 3 mm) of the 30-gauge needle should be inserted into the skin (Figs. 5.66 and 5.67ab). The dose may vary from 1–3 U Botox or from 3–8 U Dysport. In patients with a long upper lip, more superficial injections with the lowest doses should be initially applied.

It is advisable to conduct a two-step treatment in patients that are treated for the first time. After 7–15 days, depending on the result obtained, an extra dose may be applied.

Treatment of the m. levator labii superioris alaeque nasi
- One injection point per side
- Botox dose: 1–3 U per side
- Dysport dose: 2–8 U per side

## 5.7.6 Complications

Excessive blocking of the nasolabial fold may result in lengthening of the upper lip or complete upper lip drooping at one or both sides. The central and lateral incisors become excessively hidden. Partial to complete upper lip drooping, due to hypotony or atony of the central elevators may lead to excessive upper lateral pulling of the zygomaticus major and as a consequence, a 'joker smile' may result.

A more common finding is asymmetry after the injection. In static analysis, the treated area may present no problem with a nice flattening of the bulging area at the upper part of the nasolabial fold (Fig. 5.68a,b). However, during animation, the asymmetry becomes evident (Fig. 5.69a,b). Asymmetries are easily resolved with the injection of an extra dose at the side where the muscle is still over-contracted.

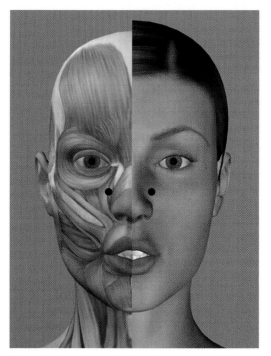

**Fig. 5.66.** Injection points for the correction of the nasolabial fold

## 5.7.7 Tips and Tricks

■ Start with the best candidates for the treatment of the nasolabial fold with botulinum toxin: young, no skin atrophy, short upper lip and gummy smile. Avoid older patients with an excessively long upper lip, flat cheeks and muscle hypotonicity during animation.

## 5.7.8 References

de Maio M (2004) The minimal approach: an innovation in facial cosmetic procedures. Aesthetic Plast Surg 28(5):295-300

Kane MA (2003) The effect of botulinum toxin injections on the nasolabial fold. Plast Reconstr Surg 112(5 Suppl):66S-72S; discussion 73S-74S

Kane MA (2005) The functional anatomy of the lower face as it applies to rejuvenation via chemodenervation. Facial Plast Surg 21(1):55-64

Klein AW (2004) Contraindications and complications with the use of botulinum toxin. Clin Dermatol 22(1):66-75

McCracken MS et al. (2006) Hyaluronic acid gel (Restylane) filler for facial rhytids: lessons learned from American Society of Ophthalmic Plastic and Reconstructive Surgery member treatment of 286 patients. Ophthal Plast Reconstr Surg 22 (3):188-91

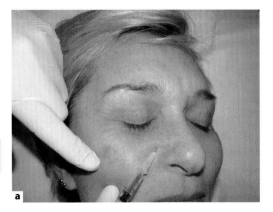
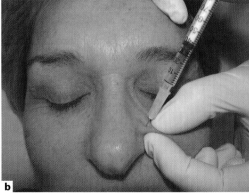

**Fig. 5.67.** **a** The injection of BNT-A should be directed at the bulging area at the upper part of the nasolabial fold. The most superficial fibers should be blocked. If the deeper fibers are blocked, upper lip ptosis may result. **b** Pinching the medial slip of the levator labii superioris alaeque nasi facilitates the correct injection of BNT-A and decreases pain

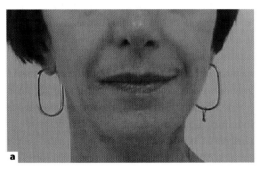
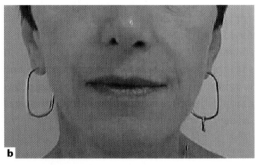

**Fig. 5.68a,b.** Before, and seven days after the first treatment with BNT-A in the nasolabial fold. The result is quite symmetrical at rest

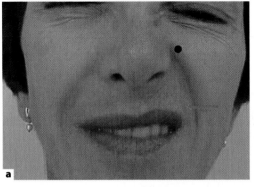
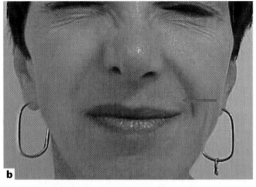

**Fig. 5.69a,b.** Seven days after the initial injection with BNT-A to smooth the prominent nasolabial fold, the patient presented an asymmetry during animation, with over-contraction of the m. levator labii superioris alaeque nasi. Note that the teeth show mainly on the left-hand side. The patient was given an extra injection of BNT-A to balance the asymmetry (see black dot)

*Mauricio de Maio*

### 5.8.1 Introduction

The use of botulinum toxin in the upper and lower thirds of the face has been carried out with a very safe profile and good reproducible results. Many studies have been published in these areas. In the mid third, however, to avoid unpleasant adverse effects, care should be taken whenever injecting close to the muscles that influence the perioral area.

Cheek lines are present in patients with thin skin and hyperkinetic musculature. Usually, they are curvilinear and are seen with advancing age in patients with skin atrophy or earlier in those people who have sun-damaged skin. These wrinkles result from a thin or atrophic skin that is submitted to repeated contraction of the zygomaticus major and risorius.

The portion of facial fat plays a very important role for cheek lines as well. Muscle traction on the skin forms more wrinkling when there is no or little fat deposit. Even young people who are very thin present cheek wrinkling that makes them look older. One of the aging aspects that compromise the face is the reduction of the subcutaneous layer. Dermal atrophy and lack of fat facilitate the formation of wrinkling even when there is no evident muscular hyperactivity. Losing weight after a certain age may be beneficial for body shape, but it can doubtlessly be an unfavourable choice for the face.

### 5.8.2 Anatomy

Hyperkinetic cheek lines result from the excessive muscle excursion of mainly the lateral and upper lateral lip elevators. Hyperkinetic lines are always perpendicular to muscle fibers; for this reason we may easily identify which muscle is dominant for wrinkle formation. Although there may be a predominance of a specific muscle, it is the resulting vector that directs the wrinkling movement.

All the mimetic muscles blend their fibers with the surrounding muscles. The cheek area is directly influenced by the m. zygomaticus major and m. risorius and indirectly by the m. orbicularis oculi (superiorly) and the m. depressor anguli oris and platysma (inferiorly, Table 5.8). As mentioned before, there are other muscles that may indirectly influence the vector forces that act upon the cheek area (Table 5.9).

### 5.8.3 Aim of Treatment

The target in the treatment of cheek lines is the reduction of wrinkling both at rest and during animation in selected cases (Fig. 5.70a,b).

**Table 5.8.** Overview of the muscles responsible for cheek lines

| Muscle | Action | Synergists | Antagonists |
|---|---|---|---|
| M. zygomaticus major | Retracts and elevates the modiolus and the angle of the mouth | All the other four elevators | M. orbicularis oris, m. depressor anguli oris and platysma |
| M. risorius | Retracts the angle of the mouth | M. zygomaticus major and m. buccinator | M. orbicularis oris |

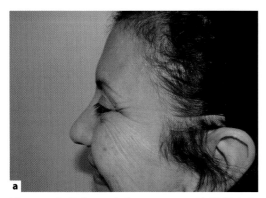
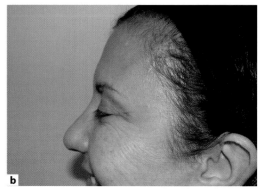

**Fig. 5.70a,b.** Before and after treatment with BNT-A for reducing dynamic cheek lines. The result should always be natural and should never impair muscle function

**Table 5.9.** Overview of the muscles indirectly responsible for influencing the cheek area

| Muscle | Action | Synergists | Antagonists |
|---|---|---|---|
| M. orbicularis oculi | Orbital part: voluntary eyelid closure and crow's feet formation. The downward extension fibers reach the cheek area. | M. corrugator supercilii and m. procerus | M. levator palpebrae superioris: for closing the eyelids M. frontalis: protrusion of the eyebrows |
| M. depressor anguli oris | Depresses the modiolus and the angle of the mouth and may produce wrinkling in the lower cheek | Platysma pars modiolus and m. depressor labii inferioris | M. levator anguli oris and m. zygomaticus major |
| Platysma | Anterior fibers: assist mandibular depression Intermediate fibers: pars labialis – depress the lower lip Posterior fibers: pars modiolaris – depress the buccal angle As it is a potent depressor, it may also influence cheek wrinkling | M. depressor anguli oris | M. levator anguli oris |

### 5.8.4 Patient Selection

Patients should be evaluated in static and dynamic positions. Static cheek lines are normally found in patients with photo-damage while dynamic wrinkling is mainly presented in patients with thin and fair skin. On palpation, the skin feels thin and fragile. Dermal atrophy should also be evaluated as well as reduction of fat content. Young patients with thin skin usually dislike cheek wrinkling because it makes them look older. (Fig. 5.71a,b) Patients with dry skin are also more likely to present fine wrinkling. Patients with oily skin usually present coarser wrinkling. (Fig. 5.72a,b)

Older patients are more likely to develop cheek lines, either from photo-damage or from dermal or subcutaneous atrophy. The presence of static cheek lines make them look even older. The best treatments for multiple fine static cheek lines are chemical peels or laser resurfacing. Cheek atrophy may be improved with fillers or fat grafts, which will interpose a biomechanical blocking for muscular traction.

During animation, some patients may present muscular hyperactivity of the lateral and upper lateral muscles; the risorius and zygomaticus major, respectively. Dynamic cheek lines can be mild and be present only from 1 to 2 cm laterally from the oral commissure or be very prominent and along the whole cheek (Fig. 5.73a,b). Static lines resulting from photo-damage or skin atrophy usually worsen during animation. Although static cheek lines are better treated with either fillers or exfoliative methods, botulinum toxin may also be helpful by relaxing the muscle fibers that insert into the deep dermis.

### 5.8.5 Technique

The most important message concerning the technique of injection into the cheek lines is that the muscular excursion should not be impaired. The muscular contraction should be slightly reduced so that superficial skin wrinkling is softened.

Usually there is no need for any use of topical anesthetics, because the injection on the cheek is not painful. After cleansing, the patient is examined in static and dynamic positions. As the quantity of lines may vary from patient to patient, the marking should also vary from a single row with two injection sites to two rows with four injection sites (Figs. 5.74 and 5.75).

The dynamic analysis should guide the positioning of the injection sites. The first and (if needed) the second row should be on the area with the highest concentration of dynamic lines. Usually the dynamic lines start from 1 to 2 cm from the oral commissure.

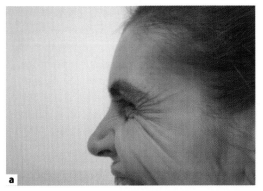 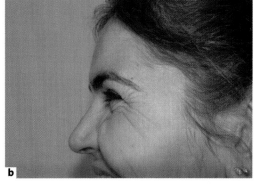

**Fig. 5.71a,b.** Typical young patient with thin skin and cheek wrinkling before and after treatment with BNT-A. A natural reduction with no complication was obtained

5

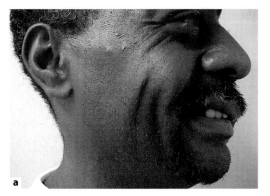
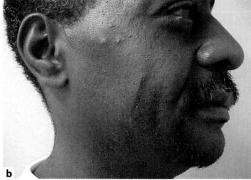

**Fig. 5.72. a** Male patient with thick and oily skin which produces coarse wrinkling. **b** Nice reduction of cheek wrinkling during animation after treatment with BNT-A

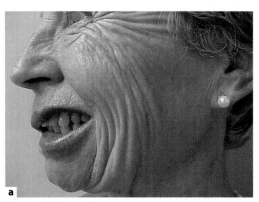
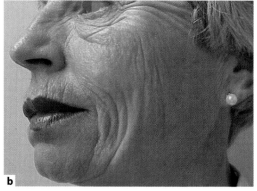

**Fig. 5.73a,b.** Patient with hyperkinetic cheek lines before and after treatment with BNT-A. Note that skin wrinkling, and muscle excursion strength was reduced. This may be considered a complex case, and a review of the section on asymmetries (Sect. 6.1) is advisable

To proceed with the marking, an imaginary line from the oral commissure to the pre-auricular area at the tragal level should be used as a guideline. The first row should be from 1 to 2 cm away from the oral commissure, and two injection sites marked 0.5 cm above and 0.5 cm below the imaginary line. If needed, a second row should be from 1 to 2 cm away from the first row, and two other points marked exactly as on the first row (Fig. 5.76a,b).

After the marking is finished, the needle should be inserted parallel about 2–3 mm into the skin at dermal or sub-dermal level. Deeper injections may result in muscular excursion impairment (Fig. 5.77a,b). A low volume and

low dose of BNT-A is also important to avoid diffusion down into the deeper muscle fibers. Initially, 1–3 U Botox or 3–9 U Dysport in total should be injected into each cheek side. If needed, a second treatment after 7–15 days may increase the dose. Of utmost importance is that a papule should be seen at the needle tip to guarantee that the injection is intradermal or maximum sub-dermal. (see Section 6.3. micro-injections)

Treatment of cheek lines
- One single row to up to two rows of two injection points per side

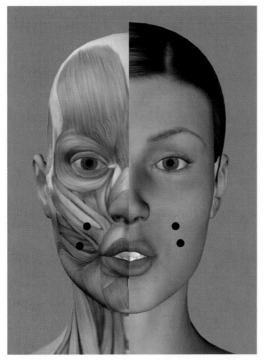

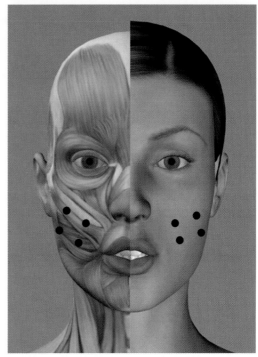

**Fig. 5.74.** Minimal injection sites for intradermal treatment of mild cheek lines. Note that these injections should not reach the muscle layers. The blocking should be targeted at the subdermal muscular fibers that produce skin wrinkling

**Fig. 5.75.** For stronger muscles, oily and thick skin, or for multiple cheek lines, the two-row technique should be used

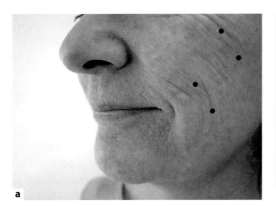

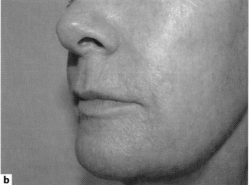

a    b

**Fig. 5.76a,b.** Before and after three sessions of treatment of the cheeks using the two-row technique

5

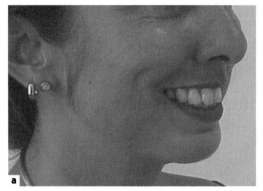
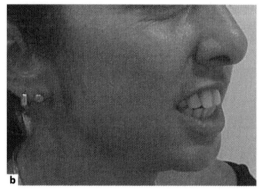

**Fig. 5.77a,b.** This patient complained about the line on her right cheek. Before and after inadvertent deep injection at the cheek line. Note that with the blocking of both the m. zygomaticus major and m. risorius, there is an awkward change of the smile line with predominance of the upper elevators and the depressors

- Only very superficial intra- or subdermal injections (see also Sect. 6.3 for microinjection technique)
- Botox dose: 1–3 U total dose per cheek
- Dysport dose: 3–9 U total dose per cheek

## 5.8.6 Complications ❗

The complications with the treatment of cheek lines include asymmetry, upper lip ptosis and muscle excursion impairment. The complications are mainly results of deep injections or the use of high doses and volume in the cheek area. With the inadvertent blocking of the m. zygomaticus major, upper lip ptosis may result. With m. risorius blocking, smile excursion may be impaired and result in imbalance of the lip elevators and depressors.

## 5.8.7 Tips and Tricks

- The cheek lines are best treated with either intradermal or subdermal injections (Fig. 5.78). Multiple treatments are usually necessary to obtain a nice result.

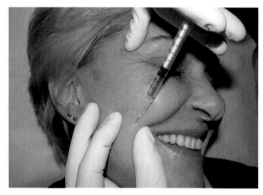

**Fig. 5.78.** The injection of BNT-A at this level should be intradermal in order not to compromise the deep fibers and impair muscle excursion

## 5.8.8 References

Bikhazi NB, Maas CS (1997) Refinement in the rehabilitation of the paralyzed face using botulinum toxin. Otolaryngol Head Neck Surg 117(4):303-7

De Maio M (2004) The minimal approach: an innovation in facial cosmetic procedures. Aesthetic Plast Surg 28(5):295-300

Ellis DA, Tan AK (1997) Cosmetic upper-facial rejuvenation with botulinum. J Otolaryngol 26(2):92-6

Matarasso SL, Matarasso A (2001) Treatment guidelines for botulinum toxin type A for the periocular region and a report on partial upper lip ptosis following injections to the lateral canthal rhytids. Plast Reconstr Surg 108(1):208-14; discussion pp 215-7

Spiegel JH, DeRosa J (2005) The anatomical relationship between the orbicularis oculi muscle and the levator labii superioris and zygomaticus muscle complexes. Plast Reconstr Surg 116(7):1937-42; discussion pp 1943-4

## 5.9 Gummy smile

*Mauricio de Maio*

### 5.9.1 Introduction

Excessive gum show during smile or laugh defines the gummy smile. From an aesthetic point of view, it is undesirable to present this type of smile. Patients usually are not aware of it and only realize it after being photographed. In some cases, it is considered quite disturbing, especially for women. Some patients are prone to exhibit this kind of smile, such as those with a short distance between the nasal base and Cupid's bow as well as those with a facial convex profile with a prominent nose and underdeveloped chin. They are mainly mouth breathers with upper lip retraction and visible upper incisors. Deep nasolabial folds are also found in these patients.

#### 5.9.1.1 Types of Smile

There are three different patterns of smile. The second most common (35%) is the one that may produce the gummy smile. It is also known as the canine smile due to the fact that it is the central part of the mouth that is elevated. The m. levator labii superioris that elevates the upper lip is responsible for this pattern of smile. If there is a natural over-contraction of this muscle, the gummy smile results. The m. levator labii superioris alaeque nasi can also play an important role in producing the gummy smile. Both the medial part of the upper lip and the nasal flare are elevated when this muscle is contracted. In patients with gummy smile it is very common to see the inversion of the upper lip while smiling. These patients are usually bad candidates for upper lip augmentation with fillers, which usually results in excessive filling of the vermillion. The best approach in these cases is a combination of fillers and botulinum toxin. The synergism of both treatments leads to a more natural look.

Other patterns can also be found. The most common type of smile (67%), the 'Mona Lisa' smile, results from the dominant action of the m. zygomaticus major. It is a strong outward pull of the corners of the mouth with a gentle lifting of its central part. The full denture smile (2%) is the least common of all, where both the upper and lower teeth are exposed.

The golden proportion establishes that the upper lip should cover the upper third of the central incisors.

### 5.9.2 Anatomy

The orbicularis oris is a sphincter around the mouth. It is a bilateral circumferential muscle that closes and puckers the mouth and forms a purse string. It anchors to the nasal septum and the maxilla above and to the medial part of the mandible below. The deeper layers of the orbicularis oris are the fibers of the buccinator and are reinforced by the incisive bundles.

From the skin, short oblique fibers traverse the thickness of the lip in the direction of the mucosa. The more superficial layer is formed by the insertion of seven small muscles: five elevators and two depressors. At the corner of the mouth, there is an area denominated modiolus, it is where the muscles that elevate and depress the lip interdigitate. The elevators consist of the m. zygomaticus major and minor, m. levator labii inferioris, m. levator labii superioris alaeque nasi and m. levator anguli oris. The zygomaticus major muscle originates from the zygoma (anterior to the zygomaticotemporal suture) and runs inferiorly and medially to the angle of the mouth and contributes to the modiolus. The zygomaticus minor muscle arises from the malar bone (behind the maxillary suture) and passes downward and inward and in continuity with the m. orbicularis oris at the outer margin of the m. levator labii superioris. The action of the m. zygomaticus major is to elevate the corner of the mouth and it has little or no effect on the nasal labial fold. It is both the m. levator labii superioris and the m. levator labii superioris alaeque nasi that create and move the middle- and the medial-most portions on the nasal labial fold, respectively.

> The m. zygomaticus major elevates the corner of the mouth and has little or no effect on the nasolabial fold.

The main elevator of the lip is the m. levator labii superioris and it arises from the lower margin of the orbit just above the infraorbital foramen and its fibers insert into the midportion of the nasal labial fold. The m. levator labii superioris alaeque nasi arises from the frontal process of the maxilla and inserts on the alar cartilage and medial upper lip. It dilates the nares and everts and elevates the medial upper lip. It deepens the medial upper nasolabial fold (Table 5.10).

> The gummy smile may result from excessive action of the m. levator labii superioris alaeque nasi and/or the m. levator labii superioris.

### 5.9.3  Aim of Treatment

The aim of treating gummy smile with botulinum toxin is to avoid gingiva showing at rest and to reduce excessive gum exposure during a smile.

### 5.9.4  Patient Selection

The patient should be analyzed in a static and dynamic perspective. The static analysis should focus on the lips and the nose. In general, patients with a gummy smile have a short distance between the upper lip and the base of the nose. The upper lip is mainly thin and the nasal labial angle is 90° or less. The upper lip is often retracted and the upper incisors are visible at rest. It is called the open lip posture.

**Table 5.10.** Overview of the muscles responsible for the gummy smile

| Muscle | Action | Synergists | Antagonists |
|---|---|---|---|
| M. levator labii superioris alaeque nasi | Medial part: dilates the nostril<br>Lateral part: raises and everts the upper lip | Medial part: m. dilator nasi<br>Lateral part: m. levator labii superioris, mm. zygomaticus major and minor and m. levator anguli oris | M. depressor anguli oris and m. orbicularis oris |
| M. levator labii superioris | Elevates and everts the upper lip | Lateral part of the m. levator labii superioris alaeque nasi, m. levator anguli oris and mm. zygomaticus major and minor | M. depressor anguli oris and m. orbicularis oris |

On animation or during the smile, the gingiva is highly visible. On the frontal and profile views, there is excessive gum show and, normally, drooping of the tip of the nose. The upper lip may also invert becoming even thinner. This is also one of the cases where lip augmentation with fillers presents an inefficient result. Patients and injectors get disappointed with the lip augmentation procedure, mainly because it results in excessive lip augmentation, leading to an unnatural look. The dynamic or muscle component which provokes the upper lip thinning is not treated.

As there are many muscles that act upon the perioral area with synergistic and antagonistic behavior, careful patient selection is mandatory. To minimize complications, one should select patients with a very short upper lip at static position and major gummy show at rest and during animation.

After 15 days the patient should be evaluated, focusing on the treatment effect and asymmetries. In the case of a partial result, an extra dose should be given, from 50 to 100% of the initial dose according to the percentage of effect obtained. If asymmetry results, one has to determine which side is still elevating excessively and an extra dose should be given to balance both sides.

> Treatment of the gummy smile in patients with a prominent nasolabial fold and short upper lip
> - One injection point per side: upper injection (m. levator labii superioris alaeque nasi)
> - Botox dose: 2-3 U (upper injection) (starting dose)
> - Dysport dose: 5-7 U (upper injection) (starting dose)

### 5.9.5 Technique

The patient should be asked to smile at maximum contraction. It must be evaluated whether the patient presents only a gummy smile or if there is also a deepening of the nasolabial fold at the nasal flare level. If the patient presents both the gummy smile and the deep nasolabial fold, the injection should be at the labial component of the levator labii superioris alaeque nasi (Figs. 5.79–5.81a-c). The injection should be positioned at the bulging area at the uppermost part of the nasolabial fold. At this level, the muscle is superficial and only the first third (+/- 3 mm) of the 30-gauge needle should be inserted into the skin and muscle. The dose should be 2 or 3 U Botox or 5-7 U Dysport at each side.

If the patient has a flat nasolabial fold and gummy smile, the injection should be done at a lower level, into the levator labii superioris (Figs. 5.82–5.84a,b). Also, a lower dose should be given, from 1 to 2 U Botox or 3–4 U Dysport. The injection at this level should be below the orbicularis oris.

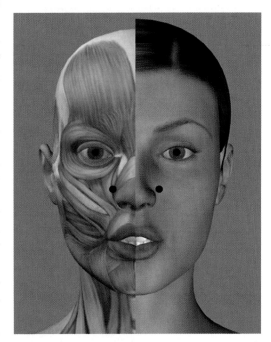

**Fig. 5.79.** Injection points for correcting a gummy smile in patients with a prominent nasolabial fold and short upper lip

5

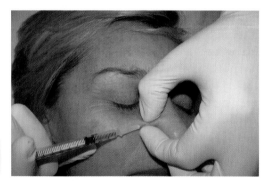

**Fig. 5.80.** The treatment of gummy smile with BNT-A may be conducted at the upper part of the nasolabial fold by blocking the lateral slip of the levator labii superioris alaeque nasi. The best candidates for this location are those with a prominent nasolabial fold and short upper lip

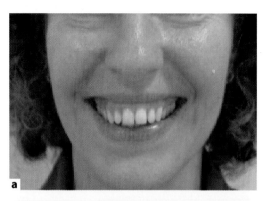

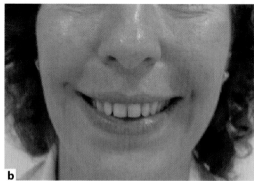

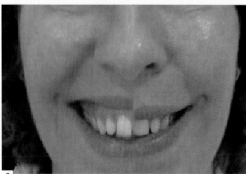

**Fig. 5.81. a** A patient presenting gummy smile before treatment with BNT-A. **b** After treatment, there is correction of the gummy show with perfect hiding of just the upper third of the central incisors. With the medial muscles (m. levator labii superioris) blocked, there is a slight tendency for upper lateral pulling with the zygomaticus muscle. There is a modification of the smile pattern **c** Split photograph of a,b, clearly depicting the positive changes in this patient with gummy smile

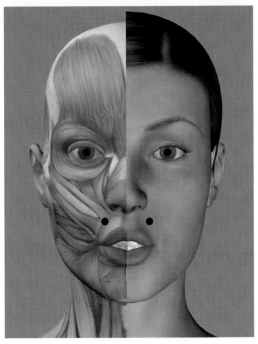

**Fig. 5.82.** Injection points for correcting gummy smile in patients with flat nasolabial folds and a longer upper lip

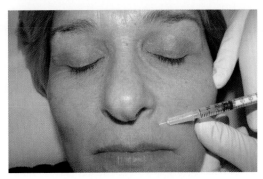

**Fig. 5.83.** The lower injection is suitable for patients with a flat nasolabial fold and longer upper lip. The injection should be beneath the m. orbicularis oris, so they should be placed more deeply. At this injection level, both the fibers of the m. levator labii superioris alaeque nasi and m. levator labii superioris may be reached. The upper lip should not be lengthened by this technique

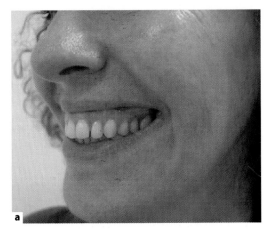
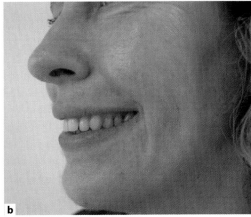

**Fig. 5.84a,b.** Excessive medial and lateral show may be corrected with the injection of BNT-A. Note that there is upper lip elongation and an improvement of vermillion fullness after the treatment. Before muscle blocking, the upper lip looks thin due to upper muscular traction and vermillion inversion

Treatment of the gummy smile in patients with flat nasolabial folds and longer upper lips.

- One injection point per side: lower injection (m. levator labii superioris alaeque nasi and m. levator labii superrioris).
- Botox dose: 1-2 U (lower injection) (starting dose)
- Dysport dose: 3-4 U (lower injection) (starting dose)

### 5.9.6 Complications

### 5.9.6.1 Asymmetries

The most common complications with the treatment of gummy smile are asymmetries and upper lip drooping. As nobody is 100% symmetric, it is important that any asymmetry should be shown to the patients before the treatment. Photographic documentation should also be undertaken.

Symmetrical injections in asymmetrical patients may result in worsening of the asymmetry. Usually, static analysis does not show any sign of imbalance; it is seen only during animation. Mild asymmetries are tolerable and should be corrected as required by the patients. However, moderate to severe asymmetries should be corrected as soon as evidenced. To avoid further complications, 25 to 50% of the initial dose should be administered and the outcome evaluated after 7–15 days.

### 5.9.6.2 Upper Lip Drooping

Excessive drooping of the medial part of the upper lip may happen if excessive blocking is undertaken. As a consequence, there is excessive lateral pulling of the zygomaticus major, and the 'joker' smile may result. A slight blocking of

the zygomaticus major may reduce the excessive lateral pulling.

### 5.9.7 Tips and Tricks

- Select patients with the open lip posture at rest and with a short upper lip. Even if excessive upper lip elongation results, it will benefit the patient.

### 5.9.8 References

Corliss R (2002) Smile--you're on botox! Time 159(7):59

Tulley P et al. (2000) Paralysis of the marginal mandibular branch of the facial nerve: treatment options. Br J Plast Surg 53(5):378-85

### 5.10 Upper and Lower Lip Wrinkling

*Berthold Rzany*

### 5.10.1 Introduction

Vertical lines on the upper lip are a strong sign of aging. Even when using injectable fillers some of these lines might still remain.

### 5.10.2 Anatomy

The lips comprise the red part of the mouth as well as the skin adjacent to it. Both parts must be considered as an anatomic unit that reaches from the nose to the chin (Salasche and Bernstein 1988). Perfect lip structure in the mucosa and skin consist of a 'V'-shaped Cupid's bow, a pronounced vermillion and medial tubercle as well as ascendant lines in the oral commissures. The ratio between the upper and lower lips, at golden proportions, is 1:1.618. A very important topographic landmark is the philtrum. The midpoint of the upper cutaneous lip is highlighted by the two vertically oriented ridges of the philtrum. The Cupid's bow is the concavity at the base of the philtrum.

The skin of the upper lip is very thin and lacks subcutaneous fat. The lack of additional support of this area together with extensive muscular movement of the main muscles may lead to pronounced wrinkles. The m. orbicularis oris is the major muscle of the lips. It has circumferential fibers that are responsible for the sphincter function of the mouth.

## 5.10.3  Aim of Treatment

The aim of the treatment is to prevent or reduce longitudinal wrinkles of the upper and lower lip.

## 5.10.4  Patient Selection and Evaluation

Treating the upper lip will inevitably lead to some functional impairment. Therefore it is preferable to treat patients with previous BNT-A experience. The treatment of the upper lip is a good preventive indication for BNT-A in younger women trying to avoid future longitudinal wrinkles.

Before starting the treatment a careful case history is recommended as the m. orbicularis is involved in more than just forming wrinkles.

For instance, patients who play the German flute should in general not be treated.

## 5.10.5  Technique

Cooling of the upper lip region before the injection might be helpful as many patients consider the treatment of this area to be quite painful. There are basically two techniques that can be combined. The injection points may focus on the central part of the lip, which is called the philtrum (Fig. 5.85) or follow the red of the lip (Fig. 5.86).

## 5.10.5.1 Technique 1

When treating the philtrum area, BNT-A will not only decrease the longitudinal wrinkles but will also flatten the philtrum area and so will reduce the landmarks of a perfect lip (Figs. 5.87 and 5.88).

## 5.10.5.2 Technique 2

When treating the area adjacent to the red part of the lip without treating the philtrum (Figs. 5.89 and 5.90) the whole upper lip might form a pout. In this case a horizontal line might appear in the area of the upper lip after treatment.

Very small doses should be used in order to avoid a dysfunctional mouth. Furthermore, slight asymmetries are quite common for this area.

**Table 5.11.** Overview of the muscles responsible for the gummy smile

| Muscle | Action | Synergists | Antagonists |
| --- | --- | --- | --- |
| M. orbicularis oris | Deep fibers: direct closure of lips<br>Superficial and decussating fibers: lip protrusion | M. incisivus labii superioris and inferioris and m. mentalis | The five upper lip levators, the m. depressor anguli ori and m. labii inferioris and the m. buccinator |

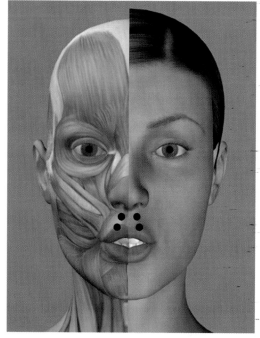

**Fig. 5.85.** Injection point targeting the philtrum (technique 1)

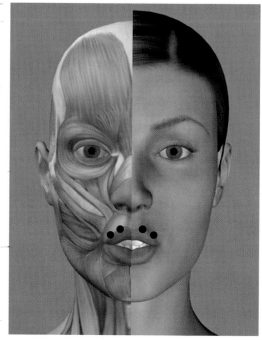

**Fig. 5.86.** Injection points following the lip red (technique 2)

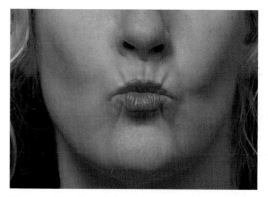

**Fig. 5.87.** Female with hyperkinetic upper lip wrinkles before treatment of the philtrum area

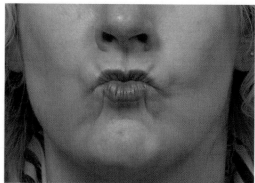

**Fig. 5.88.** Female with hyperkinetic upper lip wrinkles 2 weeks after treatment of the philtrum area with BNT-A

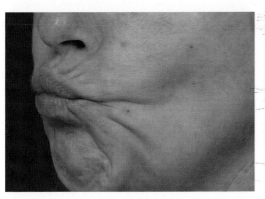

**Fig. 5.89.** Female with hyperkinetic lip wrinkles before treatment

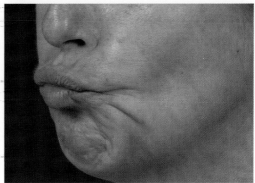

**Fig. 5.90.** Female with hyperkinetic lip wrinkles 2 weeks after treatment with BNT-A in the upper and the lower lip

Upper lip wrinkles

Technique 1

- Two or four (two upper and two lower) injection points in the philtrum area (this will flatten the central part of the lip) (Fig. 5.85)

Technique 2

- Two or four injection points along the red part of the lip (this might increase the total area of the red part of the lip and may therefore lead to a fuller lip) (Fig. 5.86)
- Botox dose: 1–2.5 U per side starting dose
- Dysport dose: 2–6 U per side starting dose

## 5.10.6 Complications

### 5.10.6.1 Functional Impairment

A relative overdose will lead to functional impairment of the lip which might significantly influence the way patients drink, eat or even speak. Patients might be unable to sip a cocktail through a straw and certain letters might be difficult to pronounce.

## 5.10.7 Tips and Tricks

- The upper and lower lip is the perfect area for the combination of botulinum toxin A with injectable fillers. Reducing the strength of the muscles will decrease the mimic wrinkles. However, it will also change the shape of the lip. Injection points in the philtrum area will weaken the philtrum. The shape of the philtrum may be reconstructed by preferably non-permanent injectable fillers. Therefore, the combination provides both: (1) reduction of the mimic wrinkles by BNT-A and (2) reconstruction of the volume and the landmark of the lip by injectable fillers.

## 5.10.8 References

Salasche S, Bernstein G (1988) Senkarik M: Surgical anatomy of the skin. Appleton and Lange, East Norwalk, CT

## 5.11  Marionette Lines

*Berthold Rzany*

### 5.11.1  Introduction

The marionette lines are important landmarks for the overall impression of the face. Deep marionette lines might give the total face an expression of being dissatisfied, sullen or even scornful. Marionette lines are a perfect target for treatment with BNT-A, often in addition to injectable fillers.

### 5.11.2  Anatomy

The perioral muscles form several strata. In the area of the lower lip and the chin, three muscles are structured over each other like tiles. Contraction of those muscles will lead to a cranky or sad expression. The most superficial part forms the m. depressor anguli oris. This triangular muscle derives from the base of the mandible and continues laterally and cranially. It inserts in the fibres of the corner of the mouth where it interweaves with the elevators of the mouth, the m. levator anguli oris and the m. zygomaticus major. The m. depressor anguli oris, together with the fibers from the platysma, drags the corners of the mouth down. This movement will induce a visible crease that descends from the corner of the mouth and gives the total face a dissatisfied, sullen or even a scornful expression.

### 5.11.3  Aim of Treatment

The aim of the treatment is to reduce the muscular strength of the m. depressor anguli oris and the fibers of the platysma and thereby induce a lift of the corners of the mouth while the patient is at rest.

### 5.11.4  Patient Selection and Evaluation

Kinetic and hyperkinetic patients are best (Figs. 5.91–5.96). Patients in whom the marionette lines are mostly due to the ptosis of the SMAS are less suitable patients for treatment with BNT-A. Here, injectable fillers are the treatment first choice.

### 5.11.5  Technique

The m. depressor anguli oris as well as additional platysmal bands can usually be easily palpated when the patient is asked to grimace. Several treatment options exist. Usually one point targets the m. depressor anguli oris and the other point the platysmal bands inserting at the lateral parts of the m. orbicularis oris (Fig. 5.97). To avoid adverse events due to the involuntary treatment of parts of the m. orbicularis oris it is recommended to keep a distance of at least 1 cm from the corners of the mouth of the patient.

**Table 5.12.** Characteristics of the m. depressor anguli oris

| Muscle | Action | Synergists | Antagonists |
|---|---|---|---|
| M. depressor anguli oris | Depresses the modiolus and angle of the mouth (e.g. draws the corner of the mouth down) | Platysma pars modiolus and m. depressor labii inferioris | M. levator anguli oris, m. zygomaticus major |

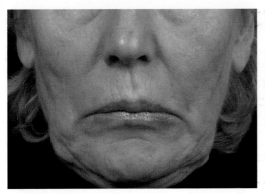

**Fig. 5.91.** Patient in her fifties with increased elastosis, grimacing before treatment

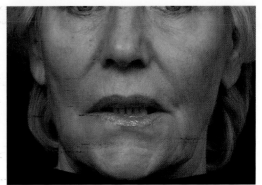

**Fig. 5.92.** Patient in her fifties with increased elastosis, grimacing 2 weeks after treatment with BNT-A

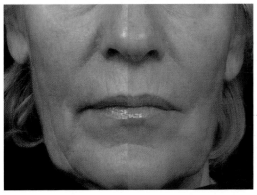

**Fig. 5.93.** Split photograph of patient in her fifties with increased elastosis at rest before and 2 weeks after treatment with BNT-A

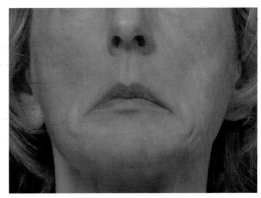

**Fig. 5.94.** Patient in her forties grimacing before treatment

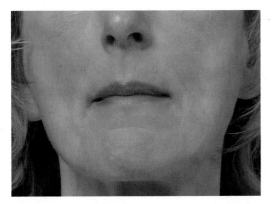

**Fig. 5.95.** Patient in her forties grimacing 2 weeks after treatment with BNT-A

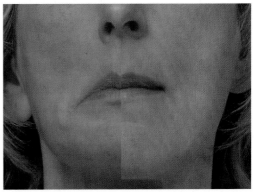

**Fig. 5.96.** Split photograph of patient in her forties grimacing before, and 2 weeks after, treatment with BNT-A

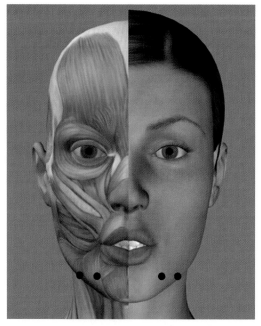

**Fig. 5.97.** Injection points for the marionette lines. Both the m. depressor anguli oris and the platysma are targeted

Marionette lines
- One injection point per site targeting the m. depressor anguli oris. The point should be at least 1cm away from the corner of the mouth. The muscle can be felt while contracted. Usually the point can be found in the elongation of the nasolabial fold (Fig. 5.97)
- Another injection point should be put more laterally in the area of the mandible in order to target the platsymal bands
- Botox dose: max. 5 U per injection point
- Dysport dose: max. 10 U per injection point

## 5.11.6  Complications

High doses or an injection that is too close to the corner of the mouth might lead to asymmetry

as well as difficulties while eating and drinking, such as drooling.

## 5.11.7  Tips and Tricks

- Like the upper and lower lip, the area of the marionette lines is a perfect area for the combination of BNT-A with injectable fillers. Reducing the strength of the muscles will lift the corner of the mouth and flatten the Marionette lines. Injectable fillers, preferably biodegradable ones, might be used to decrease these lines even more.

## 5.12  Cobblestone chin

*Berthold Rzany*

## 5.12.1  Introduction

The cobblestone chin or dimpled chin develops when the m. mentalis, which inserts with several fibers in the dermis of this area, is contracted. Contraction can be achieved by pulling the lower lip down. Injections with BNT-A will lead to a smoothing of this area of the chin.

## 5.12.2  Anatomy

The m. mentalis belongs to the muscles of the perpendicular system of the perioral area and is the most medial and deepest muscle of this area. It derives from the lower incisors and inserts transversally in the dermis of the chin. The muscles from both sides crisscross each other. While contracted, the chin may show a cobblestone pattern. In addition, the mentolabial crease might be increased while shoving the lower lip forward.

### 5.12.3 Aim of Treatment

The aim of the treatment is to reduce the cobblestone pattern on the chin.

### 5.12.4 Patient Selection and Evaluation

A patient rarely just asks for treatment of the cobblestone pattern. More often patients ask for a rejuvenation of the lower face in which the co-treatment of the m. mentalis will add to treatment satisfaction (Fig. 5.98a,b).

### 5.12.5 Technique

BNT-A can be either injected in one single point or in two lateral points, one on the left and one on the right site, approximately 0.5–1 cm above the chin (Fig. 5.99). No injection points should come closer than 1 cm of the lower lip. Although the muscle is quite deeply located, superficial injections are fine and will lead to quite satisfactory results.

Cobblestone chin
- One or two injection points, approx. 0.5–1 cm above the chin
- Botox dose: total dose 4–8 U
- Dysport dose: total dose 10–20 U

### 5.12.6 Complications

When an appropriate distance from the lower lip is kept, complications apart from hematoma are nil. Placing the injection points too close to

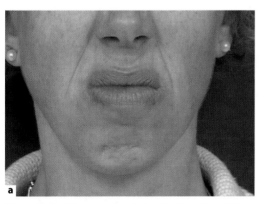
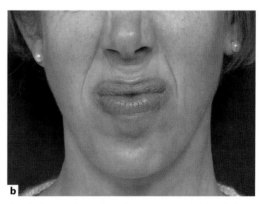

**Fig. 5.98a,b.** Kinetic patient in her forties with cobblestone chin before, and 2 weeks after, treatment with BNT-A

**Table 5.13.** Overview of the muscles responsible for the cobblestone chin

| Muscle | Action | Synergists | Antagonists |
|---|---|---|---|
| M. mentalis | Raises the mental tissue (might show cobblestone pattern), mentolabial sulcus and base of the lower lip | M. levator anguli oris and zygomaticus major | M. depressor labii inferioris and m. depressor anguli oris |

5

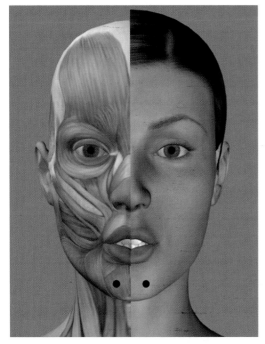

**Fig. 5.99.** Injection points for cobblestone chin

the lower lip might involve the m. depressor labii inferioris, which would lead to a dysfunctional mouth with ptosis of the lower lip.

### 5.12.7 Tips and Tricks

■ Although the muscle lies quite deep, superficial injections will lead to quite satisfactory results.

## 5.13 Platysmal bands

*Berthold Rzany*

### 5.13.1 Introduction

In slim kinetic and hyperkinetic patients platysmal bands arise when the patients activate other

mimic muscles e.g. while speaking. During aging they may become very visible forming the so-called turkey neck.

### 5.13.2 Anatomy

The platysma is the largest mimic muscle. It originates at the border of the lower jaw, covering the chin up to the angulus mandibulae. The lateral fibres of this muscle extend over the angulus mandibulae in the area of the lower cheek and also radiate towards the corner of the mouth, where they interwine with the other muscles of the modiolus. The caudal part of the platysma runs as a broad thin sheet of muscles towards the clavicle and inserts approximately around the second rip at the fascia pectoralis. The platysma does not usually cover the medial area where the cartilage of the larynx can be found.

The platysma covers the superficial fascia of the neck and is closely connected to the skin. It draws the lower jaw and the corners of the mouth down, expands the skin of the neck and extends the skin in vertical lines. In the area of the upper thorax, the décolleté, contraction of the platysma might cause diagonal wrinkles.

When treating the platysma, the close relationship to the group of supra- and infrahyal muscles and to the outer larynx muscles has to be taken into account. Apart from the diagonal m. sternocleidomastoideus, only the fascia of the neck will separate the platysma from the muscles of the larynx.

### 5.13.3 Aim of Treatment

The aim of treatment with BNT-A in the neck area is a reduction of the vertical bands that appear when the patient contracts the platysma (Figs. 5.100 and 5.101). Furthermore, lateral cheek lines and marionette lines can be improved when reducing the strength of the platysmal bands.

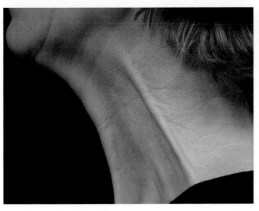

**Fig. 5.100.** Contracted platysmal bands before injection

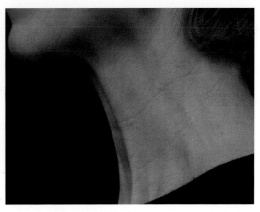

**Fig. 5.101.** Contracted platysmal bands 2 weeks after injection with BNT-A

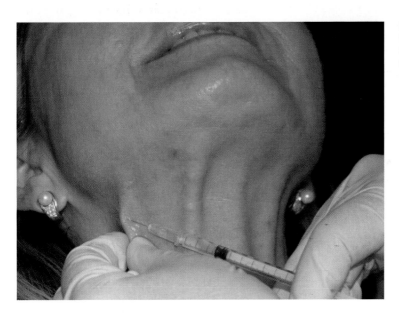

**Fig. 5.102.** Injection of platysmal bands: please note the small papules that arise after the very superficial injection

## 5.13.4 Patient Selection

Kinetic and hyperkinetic patients who contract the platysmal bands actively when speaking are best. Please be aware that BNT-A is not treatment for horizontal neck lines. Here other methods might be more appropriate, such as the combination of biodegradable injectable fillers and ablative procedures.

## 5.13.5 Technique

Patients must be in a sitting position as this is the best position to contract the platysma bands actively. Treatment follows the course of the contracted platysmal bands. BNT-A is injected every 1–2 cm. Grasping the band with the non-injecting hand might be helpful while injecting very superficially (intradermally) in the contracted muscle (Fig. 5.102).

5

**Table 5.14.** Overview of the muscles responsible for the platysmal bands

| Muscle | Action | Synergists | Antagonists |
|---|---|---|---|
| Platysma | Shows vertical bands Anterior fibers: assist mandibular depression Intermediate fibers: pars labialis – depress the lower lip Posterior fibers: pars modiolaris – depress the buccal angle | M. depressor anguli oris | M. levator anguli oris |

The pharynx region should be avoided as in rare cases dysphagia and dysphonia have been reported after BNT-A.

Treatment of the platysmal bands
- Sitting position of the patient
- Contraction of the bands by having the patient grimace
- Four to eight injection points per band, approximately 1 cm from each other (the number of injection points depends on the length of the bands) (Fig. 5.102)
- Injection technique: very superficially (intradermally) in the contracted muscular band
- Botox dose: 2–2.5 U per point
- Dysport dose: 5–10 U per point

## 5.13.6 Complications

Bruising occurs not infrequently as pressure after the injection can only be applied carefully. In rare cases dysphagia and dysphonia have been reported after BNT-A.

## 5.13.7 Tips and Tricks

- This is an area in which pretreatment with topical anaesthetics such as EMLA cream (a eutetic mixture of 2.5% lidocaine and 2.5% prilocaine) might make a BNT-A treatment impossible as local anesthetics will not only decrease the injection pain but also inactivate the platysmal bands, i.e. you cannot see where to inject.
- As platysmal bands rarely occur as single bands, treatment might become quite expensive as each band will require four to six injection points. Patients should be informed about this beforehand to avoid dissatisfaction.

# Chapter 6

# Advanced Indications and Techniques

Mauricio de Maio, Berthold Rzany

**6**

## Contents

The following three chapters will focus on advanced indications and techniques. Some of these indications and techniques may have been discussed before. However, the following chapters will offer a different view on these topics.

## 6.1 Facial Asymmetries

### Mauricio de Maio

### 6.1.1 Introduction

Facial paralysis triggers aesthetic and functional changes, with physical and psychological repercussions. Static and dynamic imbalances can affect, in a striking manner, a person's ability to express emotions. The physical aspects can bring disastrous results to a patient's self- image as well as emotional state.

A smile can express such feelings as those related to pleasure, friendship, acceptance, embarrassment, happiness, delight and/or agreement. We communicate through our smiles. Not being able to smile would be to deprive ourselves of one of our most basic tools for communication in a social environment.

Upon analyzing the half of the face not affected by facial paralysis, one can perceive the great variations in static and dynamic patterns of adaptation that the mimetic muscle tissues suffer in the absence of movement in the other hemiface.

Gaining knowledge regarding the facial nerve, the mimetic muscle tissues and the types of smiles that can be produced is of vital importance for professionals who deal with this quite complex group of patients. The expertise that derives from treating patients with asymmetries enables any practitioner to inject any cosmetic patient with excellence and confidence.

Forehead asymmetries are easily treated and are very similar to the cosmetic techniques that may be found in the specific section. Other asymmetries require more anatomical knowledge.

**Table 6.1.** Specific facial regions and the corresponding ramifications of the facial nerve

| Area | Facial Nerve |
|------|--------------|
| Frontal | Temporal branch |
| Orbital | Zygomatic branch |
| Upper lip | Buccal branch |
| Lower lip | Marginal mandibular branch |
| Neck | Cervical branch |

## 6.1.2 Anatomy

The facial nerve (cranial nerve pair VII) is responsible for stimulating the mimic muscles, creating a balance between the synergic and antagonistic forces that act upon the facial structures. It is also responsible for the muscular tonus when a person is in a relaxed state, and the voluntary and involuntary contraction of the muscles of each side of the face.

The facial nerve emerges in the stylomastoid foramen and gives origin to its many ramifications. The first ramification is the posterior auricular branch, the second is the temporal-facial branch that divides into the temporal, zygomatic and buccal ramifications and the third is the cervical-facial branch that divides itself up into the marginal mandibular and cervical ramifications (Table 6.1).

The most complex group of mimetic muscles is the one that controls the movements of the lips and cheeks. It is very important to know each muscle action and the respective synergists and antagonists when injecting patients with asymmetries in the peribucal area. The interaction of these muscles creates an almost unlimited number of facial movements and individual expressions (Fig. 6.1). There are different patterns for the smiles, depending on the muscles which are dominant. The smile may be classified into three types: 'Mona Lisa', in which the m. zygomaticus major is dominant; 'canine', when the m. levator labii superioris is dominant and 'full denture', the smile in which all of the elevators and depressors are involved. The shape of a person's smile is the result of the dynamic action of the forces that act upon the mouth, and it varies from patient to patient. A smile may also be classified as a common smile, in which the teeth are not shown, or a 'square' smile, in which the upper and lower teeth are displayed. In the former type, the m. zygomaticus major is predominant, whereas in the latter, the both the elevators and depressors of the lip are predominant.

There are five elevators for the upper lip; three of them act more on the upper lip (m. levator labii superioris alaeque nasi, m. levator labii superioris and m. zygomaticus minor) and the other two act on the angle of the mouth (m. levator anguli oris and m. zygomaticus major) (Table 6.2).

The muscles that act on the lower lip may be divided into one levator and three depressors. The m. mentalis is the levator and the depressors include the m. depressor labii inferioris, m. depressor anguli oris and platysma (Table 6.3).

There are other muscles that influence the balance of the mouth which include the m. orbicularis oris, m. risorius and m. buccinator (Table 6.4).

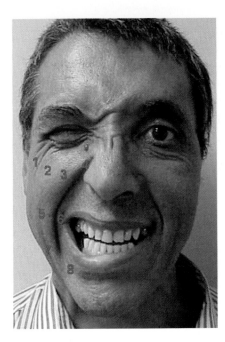

**Fig. 6.1.** Muscles responsible for severe facial asymmetries

1.  M. zygomatic major

2.  M. zygomatic minor

3.  M. levator labii superioris

4.  M. levator alaeque nasi labii superioris

5.  M. risorius

6.  Modiolus area

7.  M. depressor anguli oris

8.  M. depressor labii inferioris

**Table 6.2.** Description of the elevators of the lip, their actions and the synergists and antagonists. NB: the modiolus is the area where the muscles that elevate and depress the lip interdigitate, laterally to the oral commissure

| Muscle | Action | Synergists | Antagonists |
|---|---|---|---|
| M. levator labii superioris alaeque nasi | Medial part: dilates the nostril Lateral part: raises and everts the upper lip | Medial part: M. dilator nasi Lateral part: m. levator labii superioris, m. zygomaticus major and minor and m. levator anguli oris | M. depressor anguli oris and m. orbicularis oris |
| M. levator labii superioris | Elevates and everts the upper lip | Lateral part of m. levator labii superioris alaeque nasi, m. levator anguli oris and m. zygomaticus major and minor | M. depressor anguli oris and m. orbicularis oris |
| M. zygomaticus minor | Elevates the upper lip and assists in elevating the intermediate part of the nasolabial fold | Lateral part of the m. levator labii superioris alaeque nasi, m. levator labii superioris, M. levator anguli oris, m. zygomaticus major | M. orbicularis oris and m. depressor anguli oris |
| M. levator anguli oris (caninus) | Raises the angle of the mouth and fixes the modiolus | All the other four elevators | M. depressor anguli oris, platysma and m. orbicularis oris |
| M. zygomaticus major | Retracts and elevates the modiolus and the angle of the mouth | All the other four elevators | M. orbicularis oris, m. depressor anguli oris and platysma |

**Table 6.3.** Description of the muscles that act on the lower lip

| Muscles | Action | Synergists | Antagonists |
|---|---|---|---|
| M. mentalis | Raises the mental tissue, mentolabial sulcus and base of the lower lip | M. levator anguli oris and zygomaticus major | M. depressor labii inferioris and m. depressor anguli oris |
| M. depressor labii inferioris | Depresses the lower lip laterally and assists in eversion | Platysma pars labialis and m. depressor anguli oris | M. orbicularis oris |
| M. depressor anguli oris | Depresses the modiolus and angle of the mouth | Platysma pars modiolus and m. depressor labii inferioris | M. levator anguli oris and m. zygomaticus major |
| Platysma | Anterior fibers: assist mandibular depression Intermediate fibers: pars labialis – depress the lower lip Posterior fibers: pars modiolaris – depress the buccal angle | M. depressor anguli oris | M. levator anguli oris |

**Table 6.4.** Other muscles influencing the balance of the mouth

| Muscle | Action | Synergists | Antagonists |
|---|---|---|---|
| M. orbicularis oris | Deep fibers: direct closure of lips Superficial and decussating fibers: lip protrusion | M. incisivus labii superioris and inferioris* m. mentalis | The five upper lip levators, the m. depressor anguli ori and m. labii inferioris and the m. buccinator |
| M. buccinator | Compresses the cheek against the teeth and draws the angle of the mouth laterally | M. risorius | M. orbicularis oris |
| M. risorius | Retracts the angle of the mouth | M. zygomaticus major and m. buccinator | M. orbicularis oris |

* These muscles assist the action of the orbicularis oris in protruding the lip.

### 6.1.3 Aim of Treatment

The goals of treatment of facial asymmetries include static balance with correction of facial deviations and rotations, and reduction or total control of facial deviation during animation while avoiding any functional impairment.

### 6.1.4 Patient Selection

Damage suffered to the facial nerve may produce deformities of varying degrees, resulting in aesthetic and functional disorders in such patients. The side of the face affected by facial paralysis presents common characteristics among all patients. On the surface of the skin, there are fewer wrinkles, due to the lack of muscular traction on the dermis; the nasolabial fold becomes less evident, and there is a drooping of both the corner of the mouth and the brow. Depending on the extent of facial paralysis, and the time of onset, the aesthetic aspects may be affected to a greater or lesser extent (Fig. 6.2).

The 'normal' side or the side opposite to that affected by facial paralysis replies with a hyperkinetic reaction of the muscle tissues due to the lack of tonus on the paralyzed side. This imbalance of vector forces creates facial deviations. The dynamic deviations to the 'normal' side are less evident in paralyses that have lasted a short time. With longer periods, there are also static deviations in the labial, nasal and orbital regions, leading to shortening of the face (Fig. 6.3). It is on this hyperkinetic or hypertonic side of the face that botulinum toxin plays the most important role.

### 6.1.5 Technique

For best results and facial balance, all the main muscles on the hyperkinetic side should be treated (Fig. 6.4). The botulinum toxin should be administered through intramuscular injection with a 30-gauge needle. The needle should be inserted at an angle of 45° from the skin's surface, with the patient lying on his back. It is advisable to avoid contact with the periosteum.

The botulinum toxin should be distributed in the perioral muscles to enable the coordination of the muscles that act upon both the upper

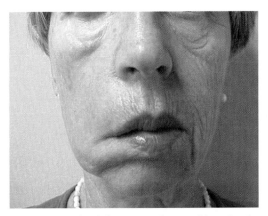

**Fig. 6.2.** Note the differences in skin wrinkling. On the hyperkinetic side (left) the muscle hyperactivity produces evident and numerous wrinkles. The lack of muscle activity results in a younger-looking skin on the paralyzed side (right)

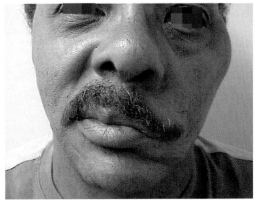

**Fig. 6.3.** The muscle over-contraction on the hypertonic side (right) may provoke facial deviations and shortening due to a long period of lack of muscle antagonism on the left side. The longer the paralysis, the more muscle over-contraction on the opposite side

6

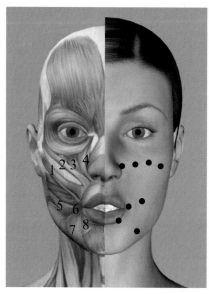

1. M. zygomatic major

2. M. zygomatic minor

3. M. levator labii superioris

4. M. levator alaeque nasi labii superioris

5. M. risorius

6. Modiolus area

7. M. depressor anguli oris

8. M. depressor labii inferioris

**Fig. 6.4.** Injection points for facial asymmetries

**Table 6.5.** Suggested injection point and doses

| Site | Botox Dose Range | Dysport Dose Range |
|---|---|---|
| M. zygomaticus major at its point of origin | 3–4 U | 9–12 U |
| M. zygomaticus minor at its point of origin | 1–2 U | 2–6 U |
| M. levator labii superioris alaeque nasi | 1–2 U | 2–6 U |
| M. levator labii superioris at the orbital margin | 1–2 U | 2–6 U |
| The modiolus, at a distance of 0.5 cm from the corner of the mouth | 3–4 U | 9–12 U |
| M. risorius 2 cm from the corner of the mouth | 3–4 U | 9–12 U |
| M. depressor labii inferioris at 0.5 cm from the corner of the mouth | 3–4 U | 9–12 U |
| M. depressor labii inferioris at a distance of 1 cm from the white line transition | 3–4 U | 9–12 U |

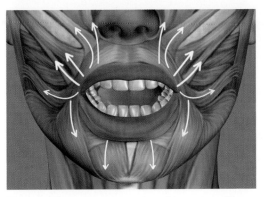

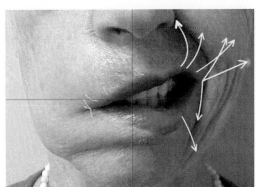

**Fig. 6.5.** Schematic representation of the vectors of forces that act upon the perioral area

**Fig. 6.6.** Schematic portrayal of the vector forces that act upon the side affected by facial paralysis, the hyperkinetic side. It should be noted that there are both straight and curved vectors, which represent the traction and rotation that the perioral region suffers due to muscle hyperkinesis

and lower lips (Table 6.5, Figs. 6.5 and 6.6). It is important to point out that the dose may vary according to the type of muscular contraction. It is advisable to start with half of the dose initially and after 15 days to add an extra dose depending on the muscular response.

### 6.1.6 Results

With the decrease of hyperkinesis after the injection of botulinum toxin, improvement in both static and dynamic positions is found. In static analysis, it is very common to achieve an excellent symmetry and correction of deviations and rotation of the face (Fig. 6.7a,b). In animation, the reduction in the hyperkinesis controls the excessive muscular excursion and corrects the excessive labial distortion and teeth show (Fig. 6.8a,b).

### 6.1.7 Complications

The adverse events with the use of botulinum toxin are generally linked to high doses of the

drug. After the injection of botulinum toxin there is an abrupt change in the mimetic muscle behavior and, consequently, in the patients' learning and adaptation patterns. Despite an enhanced aesthetic appearance, these changes may lead to functional impairment. Usually, there may be mild difficulty in speaking, chewing and swallowing. Oral incontinence for liquids and solids may happen with a high dose and misplaced injections.

### 6.1.8 Conclusions

In the treatment of patients suffering from facial paralysis, botulinum toxin may be considered as a single treatment, as a pre-operative test or as a complementary measure in post-surgical treatments. It may reduce facial deviations and rotations, minimizing aesthetic sequelae. Yet, its most important feature seems to be the potential for use in children and adolescents, who will greatly benefit from the treatment during muscular and skeletal development.

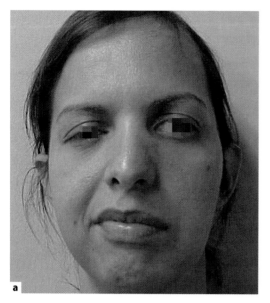 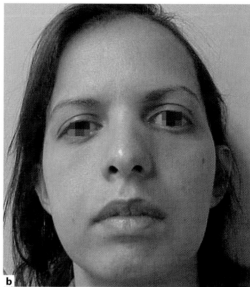

**Fig. 6.7a,b.** Before treatment, under static analysis, the patient presented a common hyperkinetic reaction on her right-hand side: a deep nasolabial fold, with nasal flare and lip deviations. After treatment, a static balance of the face is obtained. The patient reported social re-integration and an improvement in self-esteem

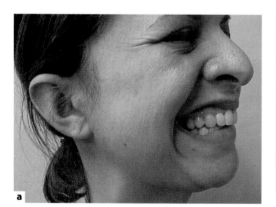 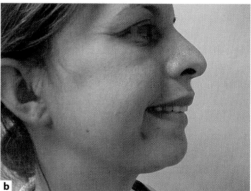

**Fig. 6.8a,b.** On animation, the patient presented excessive teeth show with distortion of the smile. After injection, there is a balance of all muscles that act upon the hyperkinetic side, resulting in an improved smile

### 6.1.10  References

Adant, JP (1998) Endoscopically assisted suspension in facial palsy. Plast Reconstr Surg 102:178

Arden RL, Sunhat PK (1998) Vertical suture placation of the orbicularis oris muscle: a simple procedure for the correction of unilateral marginal mandibular nerve paralysis. Facial Plast Surg 14:173

Armstrong MW et al. (1996) Treatment of facial synkinesis and facial asymmetry with Botulinum toxin type A following facial nerve palsy. Clin Otolaryngol 21:15

Aviv JE, Urken ML (1992) Management of the paralyzed face with microneurovascular free muscle transfer. Arch Otolaryngol Head Neck Surg 118:909

Badarny S et al. (1998) Botulinum toxin injection effective for post-peripheral facial nerve palsy synkinesis. Harefuah 135:106

Bento RF et al. (1994) Treatment comparison between dexamethasone and placebo for idiopathic palsy. Eur Arch Otolaryngol Dec: S535

Bernardes DFF et al. (2004) Functional profile in patients with facial paralysis treated in a myofunctional approach. Pro Fono 16:151

Bikhazi NB, Maas CS (1997) Refinement in the rehabilitation of the paralyzed face using Botulinum toxin. Otolaryngol Head Neck Surg 117:303

Bleicher JN et al. (1996) A survey of facial paralysis: etiology and incidence. Ear Nose Throat J 75:355–358

Boerner M, Seiff S (1994) Etiology and management of facial palsy. Curr Opin Ophthalmol 5:61

Boroojerdi B et al. (1998) Botulinum toxin treatment of synkinesia and hyperlacrimation after facial palsy. J Neurol Neurosurg Psychiatr 65:111

Brans, JW et al. (1996) Cornea protection in ptosis induced by Botulinum injection. Ned Tijdschr Geneeskd. 140:1031

Burres SA, Fisch U (1986) The comparison of facial grading systems. Arch. Otolaryngol. Head Neck Surg 112:755

Burres SA (1985) Facial biomechanics: The standards of normal. Laryngoscope 95:708

Burres SA (1986) Objective grading of facial paralysis. Ann Otol Rhinol Laryngol 95:238

Burres SA (1994) The qualification of synkinesis and facial paralysis. Eur Arch Otolaryngol Dec:S177

Carruthers A, Carruthers J (2001) Botulinum toxin type A: history and current cosmetic use in the upper face. Sem Cut Med Surg 20: 71

Clark RP, Berris CE (1989) Botulinum toxin: a treatment for facial asymmetry caused by facial nerve paralysis. Plast Reconstr Surg 84:353

Dawidjan B (2001) Idiopathic facial paralysis: a review and case study. J Dent Hyg 75:316

Dobie RA, Fisch U (1986) Primary and revision surgery (selective neurectomy) for facial hyperkinesia. Arch Otorhinolaringol Head Neck Surg 112:154

Dodd SL et al. (1998) A comparison of the spread of three formulations of botulinum neurotoxin A as determined by effects on muscle function. Eur J Neurol 5(2):181–6

Dressler D, Schonle PW (1991) Hyperkinesias after hypoglossofacial nerve anastomosis – treatment with Botulinum toxin. Eur Neurol 31:44

Faria JCM (2002) A critical study of the treatment of facial palsy through a gracilis transfer. Doctoral thesis, Medical College, University of the State of Sao Paolo.

Farkas LG (1997) Anthropometry of the head and face. Second edition. New York: Raven Press pp 545–57

Fine NA et al. (1995) Use of the innervated platysma flap in facial reanimation. Ann Plast Surg 34:326

Guereissi JO (1991) Selective myectomy for postparetic facial synkinesis. Plast Reconstr Surg 87:459

Harii K et al. (1998) One-stage transfer of the latissiumum dorsi muscle for reanimation of a paralyzed face: a new alternative. Plast Reconstr Surg 102:941

Kermer C et. al. (2001) Muscle-nerve-muscle neurotization of the orbicularis oris muscle. J Craniomaxillofac Surg 29:302

Kozak J et al. (1997) Contemporary state of surgical treatment of facial nerve paresis. Preliminary experience with new procedures. Acta Chir Plast 39:125

Kukwa A et al. (1994) Reanimation of the face after facial nerve palsy resulting from resection of a cerebellopontine angle tumor. Br J Neurosurg 8:327

Kumar PA (1995) Cross-face reanimation of the paralysed face with a single stage microneurovascular gracilis transfer without nerve graft: a preliminary report. Br J Plast Surg 48:83

Labbe D (2002) Lengthening temporalis myoplasty. Rev Stomatol Chir Maxillofac 103:79

Laskawi R (1997) Combination of hypoglossal-facial nerve anastomosis and Botulinum toxin injections to optimize mimic rehabilitation after removal of acoustic neurinomas. Plast Reconstr Surg 99:1006

May M et al. (1989) Bell's palsy: management of sequelae using EMG rehabilitation, Botulinum toxin, and surgery. Am J Otol 10:220

Moser G, Oberascher G (1997) Reanimation of the paralyzed face with new gold weight implants and goretex soft-tissue patches. Eur Arch Otorhinolaryngol 1:S76

Muhlbauer W et al. (1995) Mimetic modulation for problem creases of the face. Aesthet. Plast. Surg. 19:183

Neuenschwander MC et al. (2000) Botulinum toxin in otolaryngology: a review of its actions and opportunity for use. Ear Nose Throat J 79:788

Riemann R et al. (1999) Successful treatment of crocodile tears by injection of Botulinum toxin into the lacrimal gland: a case report. Ophthalmology 106: 2322

Rubin LR (1977) Anatomy of facial expression. In Rubin LR (Ed.) Reanimation of the paralysed face. New Approaches. St. Louis: Mosby pp 2–20

Sadiq SA, Downes RN (1998) A clinical algorithm for the management of facial nerve palsy from an oculoplastic perspective. Eye 12:219

Samii M, Matthies C (1994) Indication, technique and results of facial nerve reconstruction. Acta Neurochir 130:125

Shumrick KA, Pensak ML (2000) Early perioperative use of polytef suspension for the management of facial paralysis after extirpative skull base surgery. Arch Facial Plast Surg 2:243

Sulica L (2001) Botulinum toxin: basic science and clinical uses in otolaryngology. Laryngoscope 111:218

Terzis JK, Kalantarian B (2000) Microsurgical strategies in 74 patients for restoration of dynamic depressor muscle mechanism: a neglected target in facial reanimation. Plast Reconstr Surg 105:1917

Tulley P et. al. (2000) Paralysis of the marginal mandibular branch of the facial nerve: Treatment options. Br J Plast Surg 53:378

Ueda K et. al. (1999) Evaluation of muscle graft using facial nerve on the affected side as a motor source in the treatment of facial paralysis. Scand J Plast Reconstr Surg Hand Surg 33:47

Wong GB et. al. (1999) Endoscopically assisted facial suspension for the treatment of facial palsy. Plast Reconstr Surg 103:970

## 6.2 Facial Lifting with Botulinum Toxin

*Maurício de Maio*

### 6.2.1 Introduction

The aging process causes a variety of changes in skin, muscles and bones. Volumetric loss of fat tissue in the face produces a saggy appearance which is worsened by the gravitational forces that tend to pull the facial tissues down. Muscles respond differently depending on their position in the face: the elevators are more important than the depressors in youth and the depressors overcontract during the aging process. The elevators get weaker and weaker with time and, as a result, the vectors of forces which were antagonist to gravitational forces and were able to maintain the facial structures in an upward position, simply invert (Fig. 6.9). The depressors corroborate with gravitational forces and tend to drop the facial structures.

Understanding muscular behavior with its synergistic and antagonistic effects has enabled the development of new techniques such as 'BNT-A lifting'. When blocking the correct mus-

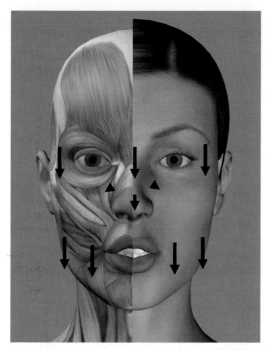

**Fig. 6.9.** With the aging process there is an inversion of vectors which, together with gravitational forces, pull the facial soft tissue down

cular group, we can again invert the vectors to an upward position, and a facelift effect can be obtained.

## 6.2.2 Anatomy: Antagonists and Synergists

To understand how the mimetic muscles act on the face, it is important to understand the definition of the prime movers, antagonists and synergists.

Prime movers are the principal muscles actively generating the movement. Antagonists are defined as the muscles that act in opposition to the prime movers and by their contraction are capable of preventing or reversing the movement. If the prime movers contract, the antagonists relax to assist their movement. It must be highlighted that this relaxation is as important as the prime movers' contraction. For example,

in the forehead, the brow elevation is only possible because the frontalis contracts AND the brow depressors relax! When promoting eyebrow elevation, we block the mm. corrugatores, the m. procerus and the lateral fibers of the mm. orbiculares oculi. Partial eyebrow elevation occurs if only partial blocking of the depressors is undertaken. Major eyebrow elevation occurs with the maximum depressor blocking possible and the frontalis with its all strength is maintained. The inability to relax the opponents will prevent the execution of the prime mover total action.

The antagonists are also important for assisting and modulating the prime movers' action. The stronger the action of prime movers and the greater the resistance encountered, the more relaxed the antagonists are. If the prime movers are involved in a precise movement, the antagonists are relaxed but immediately ready to steady or moderate the movement. Prime movers and antagonists may act at the same time. This is found in isometric contraction, for example, the contraction of the mm. corrugatores and m. frontalis when expressing concern and surprise.

Synergists are defined as fixation muscles, which are those muscles that provide a firm base for movements executed by other muscles. They are also important for providing precision and avoiding exhaustion of the prime movers. In the glabella, the procerus acts as a synergist to the mm. corrugatores for the movement of the medial portion of the eyebrows.

There are various systems for dividing the face. The classic system divides the face into three thirds: upper, mid and lower thirds. The upper third is from the hairline to the brow; the mid third is from the brow to the base of the nose and the lower third is from the base of the nose to the chin. The platysma influences the lower and mid thirds.

The upper third has only one levator which is the frontalis, whose medial fibers are stronger than the lateral fibers. In contrast, there are three or four depressors that tend to lower the eyebrow. The medial fibers of the m. frontalis have the mm. corrugatores, m. procerus and mm. depressores supercilii as the main opponents. Although the mm. orbiculares oculi may also counteract the frontalis medial fibers, it is the mm. depressores supercilii that influences this level. The mm. orbiculares oculi lateral fibers (the ones that produce the crow's feet) tend to depress the lateral aspect of the eyebrow. (Table 6.6 and Figs. 6.10 and 6.11a–c) Please note that the mm. depressores supercilii is considered by some as only a thickening of the orbicularis oculi and not as a separate muscle.

The mid third, as described above, is the area from the brow down to the base of the nose. Didactically speaking, for BNT-A lifting, elevators will be described according to their ability to act in opposition to gravitational forces. From medial to lateral, we may find the m. levator labii superioris alaeque nasi, m. levator labii superioris, m. zygomaticus minor, m. zygomaticus major and m. levator labii superioris in a deeper plane. It is also important to point out that the contraction of the lower fibers of the orbicularis oculi

pars orbitalis elevates the cheek area. The elevators at this level obey the same rule as found in the frontalis: when the medial frontalis fibers are blocked, the lateral fibers tend to elevate more for a compensatory balance. The same happens with the elevators at the upper lip level: if over blocking at the m. levator labii superioris alaeque nasi and m. levator labii superioris occurs, over contraction of the zygomaticus major and the 'joker smile' may result.

The depressors are those muscles that supplement the effect of gravitational forces. They aggravate the descent of facial structures. There are three depressors: the m. depressor labii inferioris and the m. depressor anguli oris (from medial to lateral) (Figs. 6.12a,b). The most important one is the platysma (Figs. 6.13a,b). Although the vast majority of the fibers of the platysma are located in the neck, its fibers blend with the m. depressor labii inferioris and m. depressor anguli oris: some authors even regard the m. risorius as simply a thickening of the platysma at the level of the lips (Table 6.7).

**Table 6.6.** Antagonist and synergists in the upper third

| Function | Muscle | Action | Synergists | Antagonists |
|----------|--------|--------|------------|-------------|
| Elevator | M. frontalis | Elevates the eyebrow | M. occipitalis | M. procerus, m. corrugator supercilii, m. orbicularis oculi and m. depressor supercilii |
| Depressor | M. corrugator supercilii | Draws eyebrows medially and down | M. orbicularis oculi, m. procerus and m. depressor supercilii | M. frontalis |
| Depressor | M. procerus | Depresses the medial aspect of the eyebrow | M. corrugator, m. orbicularis oculi and m. depressor supercilli | M. frontalis |
| Depressor | M. orbicularis oculi | Orbital part: lowers and protrudes the eyebrows | M. corrugator, m. procerus and m. depressor supercilii | M. frontalis |
| Depressor | M. depressor supercilii | Pulls down medial eyebrow | M. corrugator, m. procerus, m. orbicularis oculi | M. frontalis |

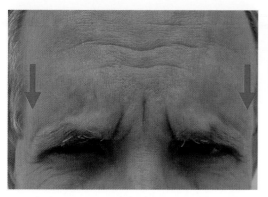

**Fig. 6.10.** Contraction of the depressors of the eyebrow provokes drooping of the forehead. It will gradually produce an aged appearance. In younger patients the elevator (m. frontalis) is stronger than the depressors

### 6.2.3 Aim of Treatment

The target of the treatment for BNT-A lifting is the complete blocking of the depressors of the upper, mid and lower face and neck as well as the subtle blocking of the medial elevators and no block of the lateral elevators. With the depressors blocked, the elevators will strengthen with time (Fig. 6.14).

### 6.2.4 Patient Selection

Patients must be evaluated at rest and during animation. Static evaluation should be directed to important landmarks of the face: eyebrows, cheeks, oral commissure, mandible and neck. The status of these structures should be analyzed (Table 6.8).

As mentioned above, the best candidates for BNT-A lifting are those who do not present significant saggy skin in the mid and lower face and neck. They are from 30 to 50 years of age and present no important asymmetries during animation. They are precisely those patients who are too young for a surgical facelift, even a minor one, but would benefit from a mild non-surgical face lift. The ideal patient for BNT-A lifting usually presents the typical signs (Table 6.9):

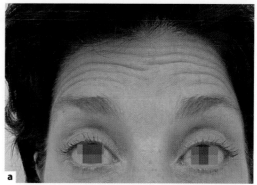

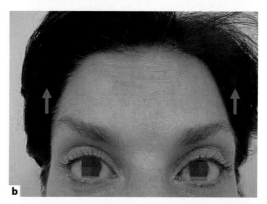

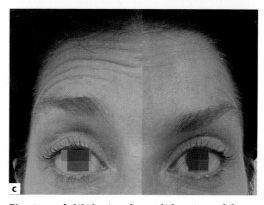

**Fig. 6.11. a,b** Weakening the medial portion of the m. frontalis and the depressors using BNT-A will make the lateral part of the eyebrow lift and erase the horizontal line in the forehead. **c** Split photograph of the patient in **a,b**, showing the effect of BNT-A after injections in the central forehead region

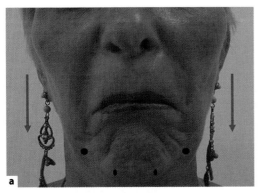
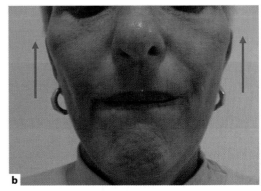

a        b

**Fig. 6.12. a** Contraction of the depressor anguli oris, depressor labii inferioris and mentalis cause drooping of the mid third, resulting in flat cheekbones. **b** After treatment of the mid third by blocking the depressor anguli oris and mentalis there is improvement of the malar projection and oral commissure

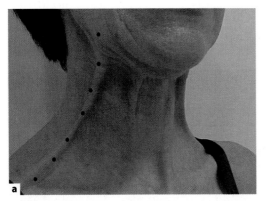
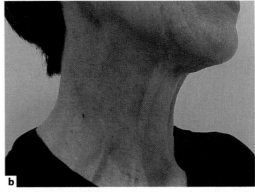

a        b

**Fig. 6.13. a** Hypertonic lateral platysmal bands distorting the mandible shape. They are pulling down the lower face, worsening the jowls. The black spots are the sites of BNT-A injection. **b** After treatment with BNT-A. Note the weakening of the lateral platysmal bands which do not distort the mandible shape. Using this method, a lifting of the lateral aspect of the face is achieved

**Table 6.7.** Antagonists and synergists in the middle and lower third

| Function | Muscle | Action | Synergists | Antagonists |
|---|---|---|---|---|
| Elevator | M. levator labii superioris alaeque nasi | Medial part: dilates the nostril<br>Lateral part: raises and everts the upper lip | Medial part: m. dilator nasi<br>Lateral part: m. levator labii superioris, m. zygomaticus major and minor and m. levator anguli oris | M. depressor anguli oris and m. orbicularis oris |
| Elevator | M. levator labii superioris | Elevates and everts the upper lip | Lateral part of the m. levator labii superioris, alaeque nasi, m. levator anguli oris and m. zygomaticus major and minor | M. depressor anguli oris and m. orbicularis oris |
| Elevator | M. zygomaticus minor | Elevates the upper lip and assists in elevating the intermediate part of the nasolabial fold | Lateral part of the m. levator labii superioris alaeque nasi, m. levator labii superioris, m. levator anguli oris, m. zygomaticus major | M. orbicularis oris and m. depressor anguli oris |
| Elevator | M. levator anguli oris (caninus) | Raises the angle of the mouth and fixes the modiolus | All the other four elevators | M. depressor anguli oris, platysma and m. orbicularis oris |
| Elevator | Zygomaticus major | Retracts and elevates the modiolus and the angle of the mouth | All the other four elevators | M. orbicularis oris, m. depressor anguli oris and platysma |
| Depressor | M. depressor labii inferioris | Depresses the lower lip laterally and assists in eversion | Platysma pars labialis and m. depressor anguli oris | M. orbicularis oris |
| Depressor | M. depressor anguli oris | Depresses the modiolus and angle of the mouth | Platysma pars modiolus and depressor labii inferioris | M. levator anguli oris and m. zygomaticus major |
| Depressor | Platysma | Anterior fibers: assist mandibular depression<br>Intermediate fibers: pars labialis – depress the lower lip<br>Posterior fibers: pars modiolaris – depress the buccal angle | M. depressor anguli oris | M. levator anguli oris |

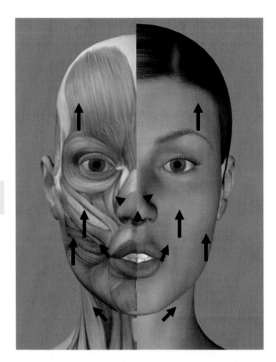

**Fig. 6.14.** The aim of the BNT-A lifting is to weaken the depressors and strengthen the elevators to promote a more refreshed look

**Table 6.8.** Desired outcomes and indications for BNT-A lifting and/or surgery

| Structure | Eyebrow | Cheekbones | Oral Commissure | Mandible | Neck |
|---|---|---|---|---|---|
| Desirable | Elevated and curved shaped with its lateral aspect slightly higher | Projected with fullness | Upward line at the corner of the mouth with a slightly projected modiolus | Well defined with no jowls and no saggy skin | No bands or saggy skin |
| BNT-A Lifting | Downwards mainly at its lateral aspect | Flat with no projection and no laxity | Horizontal or mild descent line with no saggy skin | Mild presence of jowls | Medial and lateral platysma bands with no saggy skin or fat deposit |
| Surgery | Downwards with excessive skin excess at upper eyelid | Flat with laxity and saggy skin | Very deep marionette lines with saggy skin | Saggy skin and evident jowls deforming the mandible shape | Evident saggy skin with significant laxity and fat content |

6

**Table 6.9.** Signs indicating a good patient for a BNT-A facelift

| Structure | Signs |
|---|---|
| Forehead | Horizontal lines especially during animation and none or mild lines at rest |
| Glabella | Vertical line between eyebrows mainly at frown and strong horizontal line at the nasal radix at frown. Lines can be evident at rest, but not deep |
| Eyebrow | The medial aspect at normal position or slightly low and the lateral aspect evidently low |
| Upper Eyelid | No or mild skin excess with no eye bags |
| Lower Eyelid | Evident crow's feet with no eye bags |
| Nose | Presence of bunny lines and tip droop when smiling |
| Nasolabial Fold | Prominent due to muscle hyperactivity especially at its upper position. No evident saggy skin or fat deposit |
| Cheekbones | Flat or with mild projection with no saggy skin |
| Upper And Lower Lip | Perioral wrinkling when pursing |
| Oral Commissure | Downwards with mild marionette lines at rest |
| Chin | Mild wrinkling |
| Mandible | Mild jowls presence but evident down traction with the platysma lateral band contraction |
| Platysma | Evident medial and even stronger lateral platysma bands with no or minor saggy skin and no fat deposit in the neck area |

## 6.2.5  Technique

### 6.2.5.1  Upper Third Treatment

The frontalis plays the most important role in eyebrow lifting. Its medial fibers are stronger than the lateral fibers and that is one of the reasons why the lateral part of the eyebrow drops with time. The opposite muscles to the frontalis are the depressors of the eyebrows. The mm. corrugatores and the m. procerus lower the medial part of the eyebrow while the lateral fibers of the mm. orbiculares oculi pars orbitalis lower the lateral eyebrow when it contracts.

The eyebrow lifting results from the blocking of the superior medial fibers of the frontalis and the blocking of the eyebrow depressors: mm. corrugatores supercilli, m. procerus, and the lateral fibers of the mm. orbiculares oculi. The blocking of the m. procerus plays an important role for the lifting of the medial portion of the eyebrows. Only the medial fibers of the m. frontalis should be blocked to enable the lifting of the lateral portion of the eyebrow. The mm. corrugatores, m. procerus and the upper fibers of the mm. orbiculares oculi pars orbitalis should be fully blocked. The m. frontalis fibers should only be partially blocked so that the elevating fibers are still able to promote eyebrow lifting.

### 6.2.5.2  Mid and Lower Thirds Treatment

Crow's feet should be treated with regular doses, observing that it is advisable to block the inferior medial extension of the orbicularis oculi fibers only very superficially.

It must be verified whether there is a prominent nasolabial fold and whether this is due to the hyperactivity of the mm. levatores labii superioris alaeque nasi and/or the mm. levatores labii superioris. Otherwise, injecting BNT-A into these muscles will promote no effect at all and may lead to complications. The blocking of these muscles softens the nasolabial groove. The correct indication together with precise dosing may also produce an interesting lift of the lateral malar zone: blocking the medial elevators of the upper lip will synergistically make the lateral elevators contract, lifting the lateral part of the mid third of the face, and project the cheekbones.

Patients with a short distance between the upper lip and the base of the nose are the best candidates for nasal tip lifting. If the tip of the nose drops during a smile, the blocking of the m. depressor septi nasi will produce a delicate elevation of the nose and a younger appearance.

Perioral wrinkling in the upper and lower lips should also be treated to smooth the skin in this area. If wrinkling appears only during pursing, major improvement is obtained with BNT-A. Deep wrinkling should be treated with the combination of other methods such as peels and fillers. Injecting into the upper lip medially, close to the philtrum and into the skin and mucosa transition line is advisable and the dose should be as low as possible.

### 6.2.5.3 Lower Third and Neck

The lower third is the part of the face that often shows the most undesirable aging signs, such as deep oral commissure, loss of definition of the mandible arch, and platysma bands. Blocking the mm. depressores anguli oris will lift the corner of the mouth because the opposite muscles, the elevators of the oral commissure, will enable this area to lift. The sad look around the mouth will be improved.

Injecting into the platysma may produce a better neck contour. The over-contraction of the lateral platysma bands usually pulls down the lateral part of the face and alters the mandible shape. To obtain an improvement at the mandible arch, one must block the lateral platysma bands beginning with the very upper fibers that interdigitate with the facial muscular fibers. Major lifting of the face is achieved when the lower third of the masseter fibers are blocked. As a result, the upper fibers will contract, pulling up the zygomatic zone and thinning the lower part of the face.

The dose to be used for BNT-A lifting will depend on the needs of each patient. As mentioned before, the goal is to promote full blocking of the depressors and mild or no blocking of the elevators. Below you may find suggested initial doses, which however does not mean that all the listed muscles should be injected in the first treatment. Proper physical examination at rest and during animation will identify the injection sites and muscles to be treated (Fig. 6.15, Table 6.10).

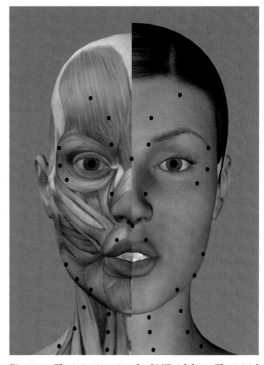

**Fig. 6.15.** The injection sites for BNT-A lifting. The initial doses should be low during the first treatment session. The second treatment should be viewed as an opportunity to improve the performance of the lifting effect

**Table 6.10.** Doses for the treatment of different muscles for a BNT-face lift

| Function | Muscle | Botox | Dysport | Comments |
|---|---|---|---|---|
| Elevator | M. frontalis | 6–10 U | 15–30 U | The blocking should be only on the most superficial fibers to remove the wrinkling and NOT its lifting effect |
| Depressor | M. corrugator supercilii | 20–30 U | 30–60 U | Full blocking is desirable |
| Depressor | M. procerus | 3–6 U | 7.5–15 U | Full blocking is desirable |
| Depressor | M. orbicularis oculi | 12–30 U | 30–60 U | The lower fibers should be injected at a very superficial level |
| Depressor | M. depressor septi nasi | 2–4 U | 8–12 U | Into the nasal base, preferably in patients with short upper lip |
| Elevator | M. levator labii superioris alaeque nasi | 2–6 U | 4–8 U | Very superficially, preferably into its medial part |
| Elevator | M. levator labii superioris | - | - | Not usually injected for this purpose |
| Elevator | M. zygomaticus minor | - | - | Not usually injected for this purpose |
| Elevator | M. levator anguli oris (caninus) | - | - | Not usually injected for this purpose |
| Elevator | M. zygomaticus major | 2–6 U | 6–18 U | Only if cheek lines are present and very superficially (intradermal) |
| Depressor | M. depressor labii inferioris | - | - | SHOULD NOT BE BLOCKED |
| Depressor | M. depressor anguli oris | 5–10 U | 10–20 U | Very important for correcting 'sad mouth' |
| Depressor | Platysma medial bands | 10–30 U | 30–60 U | Superficial if no fat content and deeper with fat deposits in the neck |
| Depressor | Platysma lateral bands | 20–40 U | 30–100 U | Same as above and the most important depressors that drop the face |

All dosages are given for the total area, e.g. both sides if applicable. The dosages are for some indications sometimes lower as described in Section 5 to avoid overtreatment.

The evaluation of results should be completely different from a surgical approach. A natural, refreshed look should be the target in the upper, mid and lower third and in the neck area. This treatment is quite suitable when patients do not have a formal surgical indication and are willing to have a quick, effective and minimally invasive non-surgical procedure (Figs. 6.16.a,b–6.20a,b).

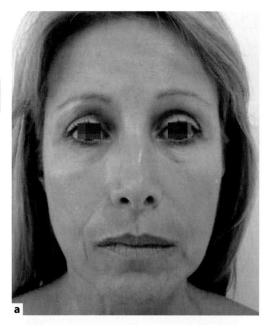

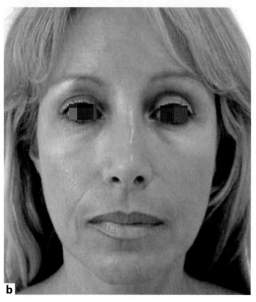

**Fig. 6.16a,b.** The ideal patient should present a tired appearance with only mildly saggy skin. After the treatment, the patient presents a natural and refreshed look

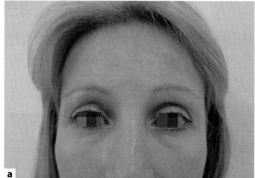

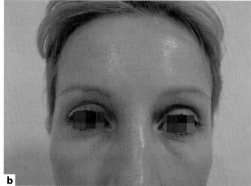

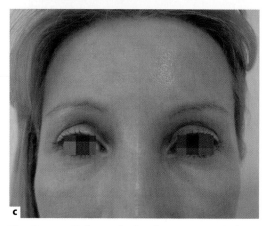

**Fig. 6.17a–c.** Before and after the treatment. Eyebrow lifting is evident as can been seen clearly in the split photograph

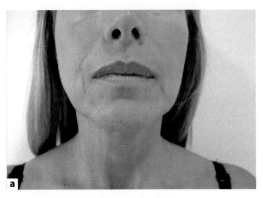 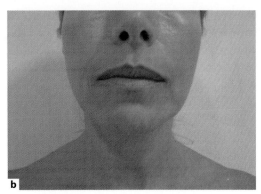

**Fig. 6.18a,b.** After the treatment, there is an improvement in the jawline and the skin seems to be tighter. There is also improvement in the neck area

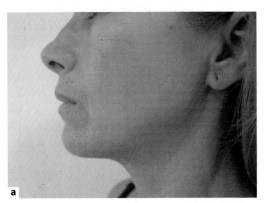 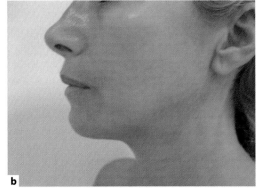

**Fig. 6.19a,b.** The cheek bone area is more projected and has a fuller appearance after the treatment

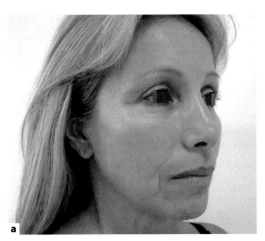 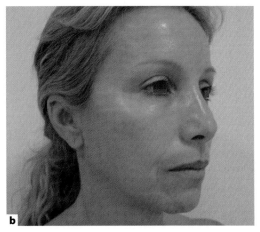

**Fig. 6.20a,b.** After the treatment there is an overall improvement in skin quality. The eyebrow is lifted, the crow's feet reduced. The zygoma area is less flat and more projected, the jawline is better shaped and the platysma bands have disappeared. Note that the result should be subtle and the procedure should not lead to a frozen appearance

## 6.2.6 Complications

BNT-A lifting is considered the most challenging treatment to achieve with botulinum toxin, not only because of the use of a considerable number of units, but also because of the areas involved. If proper static and dynamic evaluation is not conducted, unnecessary muscles may be injected and more probability of complications results.

By far the most common complication is asymmetry, due to the inexperience of practitioners in evidencing them before the treatment and injecting the site symmetrically. Another common complication is imbalance of the synergists and antagonists due to inexperience with vector forces that act upon the mimetic muscles.

Other complications such as eyelid ptosis, forehead pseudo ptosis, eye dryness, upper lip ptosis, 'joker smile' and swallowing problems are not direct complications of BNT-A lifting, but could be found in any case of improper technique to any single area. Therefore, BNT-A lifting should only be tried by experienced injectors of upper, mid and lower face and neck.

## 6.2.7 Tips and Tricks

- To ensure that no complication may result from injecting BNT-A for a facelift effect, a two-step treatment is advisable until the exact dose is defined for each patient. Generally, the depressors should be treated with a full dose and the elevators should get stronger with the absence of their antagonists' forces.
- The younger the patient is, the stronger the elevators are, and as a consequence, the easier it is to obtain a better result. With older patients, the rule is not to let the drooping muscles (the depressors) recover. In this way the elevators will become stronger and the depressors will not pull down the facial structures.

## 6.2.8 References

Ahn MS et al. (2000) Temporal brow lift using botulinum toxin A. Plast Reconstr Surg. 105(3):1129–35; discussion pp 1136–9

Atamoros FP (2003) Botulinum toxin in the lower one third of the face. Clin Dermatol 21(6):505–12

Balikian RV, Zimbler MS (2005) Primary and adjunctive uses of botulinum toxin type A in the periorbital region. Facial Plast Surg Clin North Am 13(4):583–90

Bulstrode NW, Grobbelaar AO (2002) Long-term prospective follow-up of botulinum toxin treatment for facial rhytides. Aesthetic Plast Surg 26(5):356–9

Carruthers J, Carruthers A (2004) Botox: beyond wrinkles. Clin Dermatol 22(1):89–93

Carucci JA, Zweibel SM (2001) Botulinum A exotoxin for rejuvenation of the upper third of the face. Facial Plast Surg 17(1):11–20

Chen AH, Frankel AS (2003) Altering brow contour with botulinum toxin. Facial Plast Surg Clin North Am 11(4):457–64

Cook BE Jr et al. (2001) Depressor supercilii muscle: anatomy, histology, and cosmetic implications. Ophthal Plast Reconstr Surg 17(6):404–11

de Almeida AR, Cernea SS (2001) Regarding browlift with botulinum toxin. Dermatol Surg 27(9):848

de Maio M (2004) The minimal approach: an innovation in facial cosmetic procedures. Aesthetic Plast Surg 28(5):295–300

Frankel AS, Kamer FM (1998) Chemical browlift. Arch Otolaryngol Head Neck Surg 124(3):321–3

Harrison AR (2003) Chemodenervation for facial dystonias and wrinkles. Curr Opin Ophthalmol 14(5):241–5

Huilgol SC et al. (1999) Raising eyebrows with botulinum toxin. Dermatol Surg 25(5):373–5; discussion 376

Klein AW (2004) Botox for the eyes and eyebrows. Dermatol Clin 22(2):145–9

Koch RJ et al. (1997) Contemporary management of the aging brow and forehead. Laryngoscope 107(6):710–5

Kokoska MS et al. (2002) Modifications of eyebrow position with botulinum exotoxin A. Arch Facial Plast Surg 4(4):244–7

Le Louarn C (1998) Botulinum toxin and facial wrinkles: a new injection procedure. Ann Chir Plast Esthet 43(5):526–33

6

Le Louarn C (2001) Botulinum toxin A and facial lines: the variable concentration. Aesthetic Plast Surg.25(2):73–84

Le Louarn C (2004) Functional facial analysis after botulin on toxin injection. Ann Chir Plast Esthet 49(5):527–36

Lee CJ et al. (2006) The results of periorbital rejuvenation with botulinum toxin A using two different protocols. Aesthetic Plast Surg 30(1):65–70

Matarasso A, Hutchinson O (2003) Evaluating rejuvenation of the forehead and brow: an algorithm for selecting the appropriate technique. Plast Reconstr Surg 112(5):1467–9

Mendez-Eastman SK (2003) BOTOX: a review. Plast Surg Nurs Summer; 23(2):64–9

Michelow BJ, Guyuron B (1997) Rejuvenation of the upper face. A logical gamut of surgical options. Clin Plast Surg 24(2):199–212

Muhlbauer W, Holm C (1998) Eyebrow asymmetry: ways of correction. Aesthetic Plast Surg 22(5):366–71

Ozsoy Z et al. (2005) A new technique applying botulinum toxin in narrow and wide foreheads. Aesthetic Plast Surg 29(5):368–72

Redaelli A, Forte R (2003) How to avoid brow ptosis after forehead treatment with botulinum toxin. J Cosmet Laser Ther 5(3–4):220–2

Sadick NS (2004) The cosmetic use of botulinum toxin type B in the upper face. Clin Dermatol 22(1):29–33

Sclafani AP, Kwak E (2005) Alternative management of the aging jawline and neck. Facial Plast Surg 21(1):47–54

## 6.3 Treatment with Microinjections

*Berthold Rzany*

### 6.3.1 Introduction

The microinjection technique has always been the favorite technique for some doctors. In recent years, more and more doctors are starting to use this technique in addition to the standard technique. The advantage of the microinjection technique lies in the decreased risk of adverse

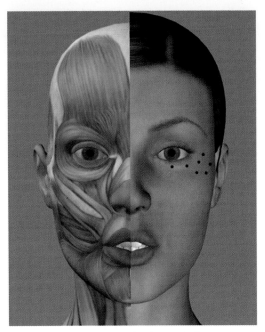

**Fig. 6.21.** Injection points for the crow's feet area using the microinjection technique

reactions as very small doses are injected quite superficially. This allows the treatment of areas like the cheeks, which for a long time had been thought to be untreatable.

### 6.3.2 Microinjections of the Crow's Feet Area

One of the first areas where the microinjection technique was used was the crow's feet area (Fig. 6.21; see also Sect. 5.4). Here the most caudal point might be very close to the fibres of the zygomaticus major, which is not a perfect candidate for the treatment with botulinum toxin A, as treatment might result in a longer upper lip.

### 6.3.3 Microinjections of the Longitudinal Lines of the Cheeks

Another example of a good indication for microinjections are the longitudinal lines of the cheeks

6

that appear when the patients smiles (Figs. 6.22, 6.23a,b). Here the muscles responsible, the m. risorius and the m. zygomaticus major are targeted. Too deeply placed microinjections might as well act like macroinjections and can cause unwanted asymmetry (Fig. 6.24a,b).

### 6.3.4  Doses to be Used

The doses to be used are the doses for the macroinjection. The only difference is that instead of three injection points, the dose will be distributed in 10–15 injection points.

### 6.3.5  Combination of Macro- and Microinjections

The combination of macro– and microinjections can be very rewarding. A good example is again the crow's feet area. Here two macroinjections 1 cm lateral to the orbital rim will effectively inhibit the activity of the m. orbicularis oculi. The more caudal area might be treated with four to five superficial microinjections, thereby reducing the risk of an unwanted ptosis of the upper lip.

### 6.3.6  Disadvantages of the Microinjection Technique

The main disadvantage of the microinjection technique lies in the multiple injections which increase the risk of punctual hematoma and the

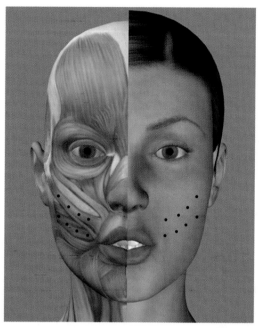

**Fig. 6.22.** Injection points for the cheek area using the microinjection technique

intensity of real or perceived injection pain. As the existing needles are not made for repeated injections, the bevel of the needle may become dull quite easily.

### 6.3.7  Tips and Tricks

■ If you use the microinjection technique, please remember the total dose you are using in this area. Otherwise you might be prone to over– or underdose.

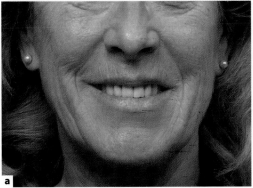 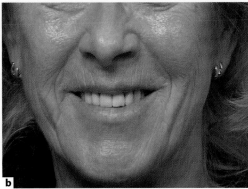

**Fig. 6.23a,b.** Cheek area before and after microinjections with BNT-A. Light decrease of longitudinal wrinkles on both sides

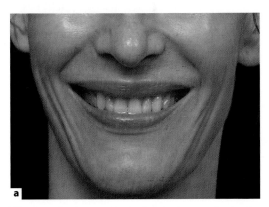 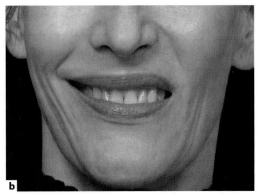

**Fig. 6.24a,b.** Asymmetry in the cheek area after treatment with microinjections. On the left side, one of the injection points was placed too close to the modiolus, leading to an impairment of the m. risorius and the m. zygomaticus major

# Chapter 7

# Safety of Botulinum Toxin in Aesthetic Medicine

**7**

Berthold Rzany, Hendrik Zielke

## Contents

Botulinum toxin is a very safe drug. In aesthetic medicine serious adverse events were only reported after using botulinum toxin of dubious origin.

## 7.1 Introduction

Although BNT is one of the most potent toxins known today, it is a very safe drug when used appropriately. Irreversible medical complications are not known and the transient and localized complications that are reported from time to time when used in aesthetic medicine mirror the reversible and localized action of the compound. Especially noteworthy is the high therapeutic index (required dose for aesthetic treatment approx. 30 U, estimated LD50 is 3000 U Botox). Serious adverse events were only reported after using botulinum toxin of dubious origin (Allergan 2004).

In the following chapter the most common adverse events of BNT when used in aesthetic medicine will be reviewed. Other indications, which might require higher doses of BNT, will not be reviewed.

## 7.2 Adverse Side Effects Due to Injection

Commonly reported side effects after BTN-injection are pain, edema and hematoma at the injection site. All these reactions typically subside within a few days without treatment.

## 7.2.1 Injection Pain

Injection site pain can be reduced by applying topical anesthetics (such as EMLA cream, a eutetic mixture of 2.5% lidocaine and 2.5% prilocaine) or pre-cooled gauze or cool packs at the injection site (Table 7.1). Please note that EMLA cream applied in the neck area will make the platysmal bands less visible.

In a small study of 15 patients the reconstitution of the BNT with bacteriostatic benzyl-alcohol preserved saline was found to reduce injection pain (Alam et al. 2002).

## 7.2.2 Hematoma/Injection Site Bruising

Bruising is reported in the BTN as well as in the placebo group in up to 40% of patients. Possible risk factors include co-medication with anticoagulant drugs, NSAID, vitamin E, ginseng, ginko and high doses of garlic. Bruising after BNT injection seems to be more common in certain areas, such as the crow's feet area. Pre-cooling of the injection site as well as manual pressure in the case of a punctured vessel is recommended (Table 7.2).

## 7.2.3 Headache

The incidence of headaches in the evaluated clinical trials varies in the BTN as well as in the placebo group from 0%–30% (Table 7.3). Interestingly, headache is not only reported after injection of BTN in the glabella but also after treatment of the crow's feet area. Headaches are usually mild and last only for a few hours (Carruthers et al. 2002; Vartanian et al. 2005). Since, according to Alam et al., up to 1% of the patients develop a severe headache lasting 2–4 weeks, patients should

**Table 7.1.** Incidence of injection pain as documented in clinical trials

| Author Year no. of patients | Drug and dose | Area of injection | % of injection pain in verum or different verum groups | % of injection pain in placebo group |
|---|---|---|---|---|
| Carruthers et al. 2003 n=59 | Botox 16, 32, 48 U | Frontal | Not reported | Not applicable |
| Rzany et al. 2006 n=221, 146 verum | Dysport, 3×10 U 5×10 U, placebo | Glabella and frontal | 0.7 | 0 |
| Carruthers et al. 2005 n=80 | Botox 10, 20, 30, 40 U | Glabella and frontal | Not reported | Not applicable |
| Carruthers et al. 2002 n=264 | Botox 20 U, placebo | Glabella | Not reported | Not reported |
| Carruthers et al. 2005 n=80 | Botox 20, 40, 60, 80 U | Glabella | Not reported | Not applicable |
| Ascher et al. 2004 n=119 | Dysport 25, 50, 75 U, placebo | Glabella | Not reported | Not reported |
| Lowe et al. 2005 n=162 | Botox 18, 12, 6, 3 U, placebo | Crow's feet | Not reported | Not reported |
| Baumann et al. 2003 n=20 | Myobloc 500 U, placebo | Crow's feet | Not reported | Not reported |

**Table 7.2.**  Incidence of hematoma/injection site bruising

| Author Year no. of patients | Drug and dose | Area of injection | % of hematoma in verum or different verum groups | % of hematoma in placebo group |
|---|---|---|---|---|
| Carruthers et al. 2003 n=59 | Botox 16, 32, 48 U | Frontal | 10%, 5.3%, 15% | Not applicable |
| Rzany et al. 2006 n=221 | Dysport, 3×10 U 5×10 U, placebo | Glabella and frontal | Not reported | Not reported |
| Carruthers et al. 2005a n=80 | Botox 10, 20, 30,40 U | Glabella and frontal | Not reported | Not applicable |
| Carruthers et al. 2002 n=264 | Botox 20 U, placebo | Glabella | Not reported | Not reported |
| Carruthers et al. 2005b n=80 | Botox 20, 40, 60, 80 U | Glabella | 5%, 0%, 0%, 0% | Not applicable |
| Ascher et al. 2004 n=119 | Dysport 25, 50, 75 U, placebo | Glabella | 0%, 3%, 0% | 5.8% |
| Lowe et al. 2005 n=162 | Botox 18, 12, 6, 3 U, placebo | Crow's feet | 18.2%, 9.7%, 6.1%, 3.0% | 12.5% |
| Baumann et al. 2003 n=20 | Myobloc 500 U, placebo | Crow's feet | 25% | 40% |

**Table 7.3.**  Incidence of headache

| Author Year No. of patients | Drug and dose | Area of injection | % of headache in verum or different verum groups | % of headache in placebo group |
|---|---|---|---|---|
| Carruthers et al. 2003 n=59 | Botox 16, 32, 48 U | Frontal | 20%, 15.8%, 30% | Not applicable |
| Rzany et al. 2006 n=221 | Dysport, 3×10 U 5×10 U, placebo | Glabella and frontal | 2.7 | 2.7 |
| Carruthers et al. 2005 n=80 | Botox 10, 20, 30, 40 U | Glabella and frontal | 20%, 15%, 5%, 5% | Not applicable |
| Carruthers et al. 2002 n=264 | Botox 20 U, placebo | Glabella | 15.3% | 15% |
| Carruthers et al. 2005 n=80 | Botox 20, 40, 60, 80 U | Glabella | 0%, 15%, 0%, 0% | Not applicable |
| Ascher et al. 2004 n=119 | Dysport 25, 50, 75 U, placebo | Glabella | 3%, 3%, 0% | 0% |
| Lowe et al. 2005 n=162 | Botox 18, 12, 6, 3 U, placebo | Crow's feet | 6.1%, 3.2%, 6.1%, 12.1% | 3.1% |
| Baumann et al. 2003 n=20 | Myobloc 500 U, placebo | Crow's feet | 25% | 20% |

be informed about the possibility of idiosyncratic severe headaches (Alam et al. 2002). On the other hand, the results of some studies point to a decrease in headache occurrence after repeated BNT treatment. However, these results were not significant (Carruthers et al. 2004).

## 7.2.4  Localized Skin Dryness

One study found an incidence of localized skin dryness in 3.8% of the patients and therefore recommended the use of skin moisturizers for treated areas (Bulstrode et al. 2002). Localized dryness could be explained by a decrease of sweat gland activity. However, in the experience of the authors, localized skin dryness is usually not a complaint.

## 7.3  Adverse Events Due to Local Diffusion/Distribution

Typical adverse events are those caused by local diffusion of BNT into areas not meant to be treated. Several of the adverse events described here have already been discussed in the previous chapters.

## 7.3.1  Eyelid Ptosis

Here, the most well-known adverse event is the eyelid ptosis which is caused by the diffusion of the BNT into the levator palpebrae muscles (see Fig. 5.23 in Sect. 5.2 on the treatment of the glabella).

Injections into the orbicularis oculi, corrugator supercilii and procerus muscles have the highest risk of producing lid ptosis. Lid ptosis usually manifests within two to seven days and can last for weeks. Using Botox in the glabella area, Carruthers and colleagues reported a lid ptosis rate of 5.4% in their first large placebo-controlled study (Carruthers et al. 2002), declining to 1.0% in a subsequent study (Carruthers et al. 2003). In their most recent studies no lid ptosis occurred after treatment of 160 patients (Carruthers et al. 2005a; Carruthers et al. 2005b). The same results were obtained from a 102-patient study, where no case of ptosis was reported after treatment of the glabella area with 25, 50, or 75 U Dysport (Ascher et al. 2004). In the German study, only one case of eyelid ptosis was reported among 127 patients, in one patient treated with 50 Dysport U (Rzany et al. 2006).

Apraclonidine, an α2-adrenergic agonist, can be used to decrease the severity of lid ptosis by stimulating the Mueller's muscle; thus an elevation of the upper eyelid of about 1–3 mm can be obtained. The most common dosing scheme for apraclonidine 0.5% eye drops is one or two drops up to three times daily into the affected eye until ptosis resolves. Similar agents for the treatment of ptosis include brimonidine (0.1% or 0.2%) and neosynephrine hydrochloride (2.5%) (Scheinfeld 2005).

## 7.3.2  Ectropion

BNT injections placed around the lower eyelid can affect the function of the orbicularis oculi muscle and lead to ectropion, causing corneal damage through desiccation. Potential risk factors are lower eyelid surgery or a higher age of patient.

## 7.3.3  Strabismus

Transient strabismus may be observed after misplaced lateral (crows feet) or medial (bunny lines) periorbital treatment. If an ectropion occurs, an ophthalmological consultation is advisable to assist in accurate diagnosis and in establishing a treatment plan.

### 7.3.4 Pseudoherniation

In patients with lax septal support, pseudoherniation of infraorbital fat pads might occur after infraorbital treatment with BNT (Paloma et al. 2001; see Fig. 5.50a,b in Sect. 5.4 on crow's feet). A ptosis of the upper lip can occur if fibers of the zygomaticus major are affected following lateral periorbital treatment (Figs. 7.1 and 7.2).

### 7.3.5 Complications After Perioral and Neck Treatment

Perioral complications after treatment of nasolabial folds and radial perioral lines include upper lip weakness.

Temporary dysphagia and hoarseness have been documented especially in older patients after treatment of the platysmal bands. In an early study, Matarasso and colleagues reported an incidence of 10% mild and transient cervical discomfort, 1% neck weakness and 0.05% clinically significant dysphagia in treated patients (Matarasso et al. 2001).

### 7.4 Adverse Events Due to Hyperactivity of Adjacent Muscles/Brow Malposition

Reducing the muscle activity in one area can lead to an overcompensation of muscles in adjacent regions. A typical example includes the effect known as the Mephisto sign, a quizzical look, Spock's eyebrow, a sinister look or 'joker' face when treating the central parts of the forehead. Paralysis of the medial parts of the eyebrows combined with a compensated hyperactivity of the lateral frontalis muscle leads to typical lateral raised eyebrows, making a following touch-up treatment necessary.

In some patients the Mephisto sign might be a visual impression that does not reflect a real overcompensation of muscles. In these cases the glabella area is lowered after treatment of the m. procerus and the mm. corrugatores (see Fig. 5.1 in Sect. 5.1 on forehead treatment).

In addition, in some patients localized muscular spasms might occur (Cote et al. 2005).

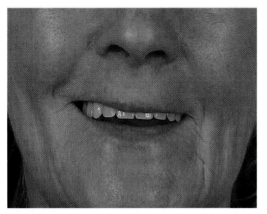

**Fig. 7.1.** Ptosis of the upper lip due to impairment of the m. zygomaticus major following injection of the crow's feet area

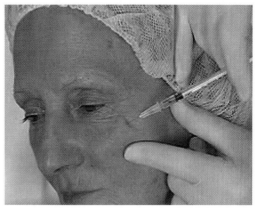

**Fig. 7.2.** Injection point in the crow's feet area that provoked the upper lip ptosis

**7**

## 7.5 Adverse Events due to Generalized Distribution

BNT, even when injected locally, can be distributed over the whole body. In contrast to other indications, generalized adverse events are reported very rarely in aesthetic medicine, where only very low doses of BTN are used.

Dependent on the BTN dose and the number of muscles injected, the onset of systemic reactions typically occurs within 1 week and they continue for 1–2 weeks. These anticholinergic effects remain peripheral since the BNT is unable to penetrate the blood-brain-barrier into the central nervous system. Typical effects of systemic BNT actions would include dry mouth, red eyes, accommodation disturbance and gastrointestinal symptoms. So far it seems that such generalized adverse events are more common for BNT-B than for BNT-A (Dressler et al. 2003).

## 7.6 Allergies to Botulinum Toxin-A

There are hardly any reports about hypersensitivity or allergic responses after aesthetic BNT treatments. LeWitt describes a persistent rash at the facial injection site (LeWitt et al. 1997). Cote reports about two cases of allergic reactions filed to the US FDA between 12/1989 and 5/2003 after use of BNT-A for cosmetic indications (Cote et al. 2005).

Although the reported data is quite scarce and not very detailed, the German package label for e.g. Botox states that reports about anaphylactic reactions have also been forwarded to the manufacturer and therefore appropriate precautions are recommended.

## 7.7 Formation of Antibodies

Formation of antibodies against the toxin will lead to a decreased efficiency due to an inactivation of BNT. In the literature, Carruthers and colleagues investigated antibody levels in 405 patients treated up to three times with 20 U Botox (Carruthers et al. 2004). In 235 patients who completed the follow-up, antibodies were found in 1.1%–1.4% of the samples which could be evaluated. However, in no case did the presence of antibodies lead to a decrease in drug efficiency.

A higher dose implicates a greater risk of inducing antibodies; in aesthetic medicine where usually very low doses are used, the problem of neutralizing antibodies seems to be negligible (Consensus Conference 1991).

## 7.9 References

Alam M, Dover JS, Arndt KA (2002) Pain associated with injection of botulinum A exotoxin reconstituted using isotonic sodium chloride with and without preservative: a double-blind, randomized controlled trial. Arch Dermatol 138(4):510–4

Alam M, Arndt KA, Dover JS (2002) Severe, intractable headache after injection with botulinum a exotoxin: report of 5 cases. J Am Acad Dermatol 46(1):62–5

Allergan Inc. (2004) Press release: http://www.shareholder.com/agn/ReleaseDetail.cfm?ReleaseID=150344

Ascher B, Zakine B, Kestemont P, Baspeyras M, Bougara A, Santini J (2004) A multicenter, randomized, double-blind, placebo-controlled study of efficacy and safety of 3 doses of botulinum toxin A in the treatment of glabellar lines. J Am Acad Dermatol 51(2):223–33

Baumann L, Slezinger A, Vujevich J, Halem M, Bryde J, Black L, Duncan R (2003) A double-blinded, randomized, placebo-controlled pilot study of the safety and efficacy of Myobloc (botulinum toxin type B)-purified neurotoxin complex for the treatment of crow's feet: a double-blinded, placebo-controlled trial. Dermatol Surg 29(5):508–15

Bulstrode NW, Grobbelaar AO (2002) Long-term prospective follow-up of botulinum toxin treatment for facial rhytides. Aesthetic Plast Surg 26(5):356–9

Carruthers A, Carruthers J, Said S (2005a) Dose-ranging study of botulinum toxin type A in the treatment of glabellar rhytids in females. Dermatol Surg 31(4):414–22; discussion p 422

Carruthers A, Carruthers J (2005b) Prospective, double-blind, randomized, parallel-group, dose-ranging study of botulinum toxin type A in men with glabellar rhytids. Dermatol Surg 31(10):1297–303

Carruthers A, Carruthers J, Cohen J (2003) A prospective, double-blind, randomized, parallel-group, dose-ranging study of botulinum toxin type A in female subjects with horizontal forehead rhytides. Dermatol Surg 29(5):461–7

Carruthers A, Carruthers J, Lowe NJ, Menter MA, Gibson J, Nordquist M, Mordaunt J (2004) One-year, randomised, multicenter, two-period study of the safety and efficacy of repeated treatments with botulinum toxin type A in patients with glabellar lines. J Clin Res(7):1–20

Carruthers J, Lowe NJ, Menter MA, Gibson J, Nordquist M, Mordaunt J, Walker P, Eadie N (2002) A multicenter, double-blind, randomized, placebo-controlled study of the efficacy and safety of botulinum toxin type A in the treatment of glabellar lines. J Am Acad Dermatol 46(6):840–9

Carruthers J, Lowe NJ, Menter MA, Gibson J, Eadie N (2003) Double-blind, placebo-controlled study of the safety and efficacy of botulinum toxin type A for patients with glabellar lines. Plast Reconstr Surg 112(4):1089–98

Consensus Conference (1991) Clinical use of botulinum toxin. National Institutes of Health Consensus Development Conference Statement, November 12–14, 1990. Arch Neurol 48(12):1294–8

Cote T, Mohan AK, Polder JA, Walton MK, Braun MM (2005) Botulinum toxin type A injections: adverse events reported to the US Food and Drug Administration in therapeutic and cosmetic cases. J Am Acad Dermatol 53(3):407–15

Dressler D, Benecke R (2003) Autonomic side effects of botulinum toxin type B treatment of cervical dystonia and hyperhidrosis. Eur Neurol 49(1):34–8

LeWitt PA, Trosch RM (1997). Idiosyncratic adverse reactions to intramuscular botulinum toxin type A injection. Mov Disord 12(6):1064–7

Lowe NJ, Ascher B, Heckmann M, Kumar C, Fraczek S, Eadie N (2005) Double-blind, randomized, placebo-controlled, dose-response study of the safety and efficacy of botulinum toxin type A in subjects with crow's feet. Dermatol Surg 31(3):257–62

Matarasso SL, Matarasso A (2001) Treatment guidelines for botulinum toxin type A for the periocular region and a report on partial upper lip ptosis following injections to the lateral canthal rhytids. Plast Reconstr Surg 108(1):208–14; discussion pp 215–7

Paloma V, Samper A (2001) A complication with the aesthetic use of Botox: herniation of the orbital fat. Plast Reconstr Surg 107(5):1315

Rzany B, Ascher B, Fratila A, Monheit GD, Talarico S, Sterry W (2006) Efficacy and safety of 3- and 5-injection patterns (30 and 50 U) of botulinum toxin A (Dysport) for the treatment of wrinkles in the glabella and the central forehead region. Arch Dermatol 142(3):320–6

Scheinfeld N (2005) The use of apraclonidine eyedrops to treat ptosis after the administration of botulinum toxin to the upper face. Dermatol Online J 11(1):9

Vartanian, AJ, Dayan SH (2005) Complications of botulinum toxin A use in facial rejuvenation. Facial Plast Surg Clin North Am 13(1):1–10

# Chapter 8

# Combination Therapy – The Microlift Procedure

8

Mauricio de Maio

## Contents

## 8.1 Introduction

Facial aging is recognized as a loss of volume (loss of underlying soft tissue support), increasing skin wrinkling, and skin folding. Age, sun damage, tobacco and alcohol use, trauma, and poor nutrition all contribute jointly to facial aging, but it is chronic sun exposure that causes the most significant skin changes. Over time, skin becomes progressively thinner, drier, less elastic, and less resilient, and as a result of the loss of elasticity, facial skin becomes more lax. Wrinkles form, and jowls are created by ptosis of the facial portion of the platysma muscle and an altered distribution of fat under the chin.

Many procedures are available for patients seeking treatment to reduce the appearance of facial wrinkles and folds; namely ablative treatments such as chemical peels and laser resurfacing, injections with BNT-A and fillers as well as facelifts. Patients desiring to re-establish their jaw lines may benefit from neck liposuction. Each of these techniques is effective in reducing certain signs of facial aging. However, each of these techniques have limitations and disadvantages, especially for the patient who wants to see an immediate improvement with minimal discomfort and time away from social and work engagements. Based on the above, it is easy to understand that a single procedure will not be able to solve the complexity of the facial changes that happen with time. Combination therapy is and always will be the best solution for dealing with different facial alterations. A facelift in a woman with severe photo-damage without any resurfacing treatment will lead to an old woman with an excessively pulled face!

> Combination therapy is and always will be the best solution for dealing with different facial alterations.

## 8.2 Botulinum Toxin and Chemical Peels

Photodamage is the primary trigger for extrinsic aging. It results from cumulative exposure to ultraviolet light and is responsible for many unwanted aging signs. The most common clinical signs include aging spots on a shallow colored skin, keratoses, static rhytids, telangiectasia and loss of elasticity. The degree of photodamage varies from patient to patient and can be mild, moderate or severe. Fillers and botulinum toxin alone will not be able to solve every skin wrinkle. The best way to reduce static wrinkling is through ablative methods such as chemical peels. Skin renewal and collagen remodeling improves the appearance of photo-damaged skin. With dermal thickening, less wrinkling appears due to muscle traction onto the skin.

The fact that superficial skin wrinkling may be treated with chemical peels does not mean that dynamic wrinkles should not be treated. Both methods should be used together to allow better results. Why combine BNT-A and chemical peels? Because the BNT-A treats dynamic wrinkles, and the chemical peels treat superficial skin wrinkling and pigmentation. Many people with sun exposure develop hyperpigmentation and crow's feet. They are the ideal patients to be submitted to a light peel and BNT-A treatment (Fig. 8.1a,b).

## 8.3 Botulinum Toxin and Laser Resurfacing

Laser resurfacing is another effective ablative method for the treatment of static rhytids. The two most common applications are the $CO_2$ and Erbium lasers. The $CO_2$ laser, in contrast to the Erbium laser, will produce more collateral thermal damage and will coagulate bleedings. $CO_2$ lasers are used like deep chemical peels against severe photodamage. Erbium lasers are used like medium peels. Erbium lasers will lead to less swelling and redness. Both of them are effective in promoting inflammation that leads to collagen remodeling and finally to a thicker dermis. Muscle traction on a thicker dermis will produce less wrinkling.

BNT-A plays an amazing role with resurfacing methods. If there is no excessive muscle movement, collagen remodelling will proceed in a smoother fashion and will probably decrease the risk of hypertrophic scars. Also, the absence of excessive muscle contraction avoids rewrinkling.

When combining laser resurfacing and BNT-A, the injection of the botulinum toxin should be performed 1 or 2 weeks before the procedure. The concomitant injection of BNT-A, and the immediate use of lasers after, especially $CO_2$, may not be advisable. Excessive thermal heating may alter the BNT-A molecule and inactivation may result. Although the layers of treatment in both methods are not the same, the immediate resulting edema after laser application may also alter BNT-A activity. So, the injection may be conducted before laser treatment or when edema subsides. The combination of BNT-A and lasers is recommended, since otherwise, even with a very deep and effective partial dermal removal, patients will still produce dynamic wrinkling (Fig. 8.2a,b).

## 8.4 Botulinum Toxin and Fillers

The combination of BNT-A with fillers is one of the most interesting non-surgical cosmetic procedures. It leads to no downtime and generally nobody can tell what has been done. It is the perfect treatment for male patients (Fig. 8.3a,b).

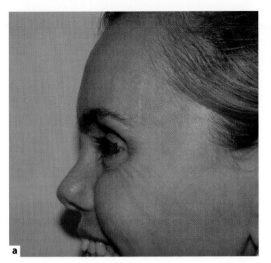
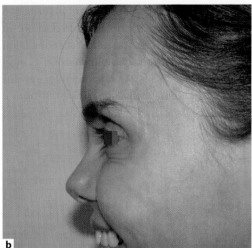

**Fig. 8.1a,b.** Crow's feet area before and after combination treatment of BNT-A injection with a light chemical peel. Please note the nice wrinkling reduction and the lightening of the skin

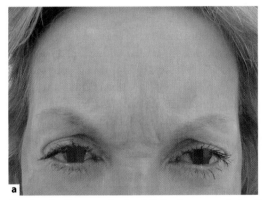
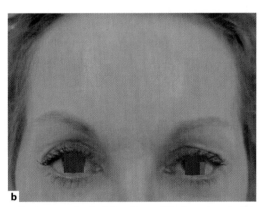

**Fig. 8.2a,b.** One month after full face laser resurfacing the patient was again depicting lines while frowning. As this would jeopardize the resurfacing result the patient was treated with BNT-A in the glabella area. After BNT-A treatment there is no visual line formation during frowning. This case demonstrated the usefulness of the combination of BNT-A with ablative procedures

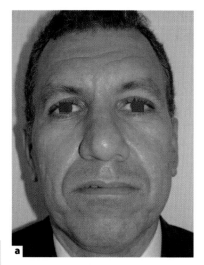
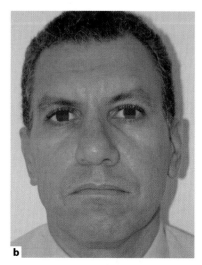

**Fig. 8.3a,b.** Patient presenting with acne scars and deep dynamic wrinkles in the forehead and glabella area. Also, a slight asymmetry in his upper lip on the right side can be noticed. Before and after treatment with a combination of injectable fillers and BNT-A. The result is very natural and there is no evidence of any cosmetic procedure done in this male patient

Very superficial and superficial skin wrinkling is best treated with ablative methods, such as lasers or chemical peels. However, medium or deep wrinkles and folds are ideally treated with fillers. Depending on the depth of a wrinkle or fold, the appropriate filler should be chosen. Why combine BNT-A and fillers? If we analyze the negative cosmetic landmarks of the face, we may notice that some of the most evident wrinkling occurs on the area where mimic activity is the greatest. The kinetics of mimetic muscles and skin atrophy determine how BNT-A and/or fillers are used. Muscles do produce more intense skin wrinkling when the skin is thin or atrophic. The single use of fillers to increase the dermal thickness may be enough to decrease the mimetic action on the skin. Hyperkinetic or hypertonic patients, however, will continue to move the dermis even when it is thick. In these patients the durability of a biodegradable injectable filler might be shorter. By blocking the muscular activity or even hyperactivity, BNT-A will directly reduce the degradation of the biodegradable filler and so prolong the duration of the effect.

Depending on the area of treatment, the decision regarding the timing of injection of BNT-A or use of fillers may differ. Usually, the dynamic component should be treated before the static component of the wrinkle, mainly because the use of BNT-A may be enough for resolving the hyperkinetic line. However, in selected cases, dermal atrophy or deep static lines do not disappear after BNT-A injection. These patients usually get disappointed with BNT-A alone and the experienced injector should recommend the concomitant use of fillers in those patients. In more complicated areas, such as in perioral wrinkling or the nasolabial fold, fillers are best scheduled to be injected first. If, after the filler injection, many wrinkles are still evident during animation, the subsequent injection of BNT-A should be considered.

Experienced practitioners may know firsthand that combined use of fillers and BNT-A will be necessary and can do both in the same session. One procedure does not interfere with the other because both are injected into different layers. Usually, BNT-A will be injected first and fillers soon after (Table 8.1).

**Table 8.1.** Combination of BNT-A with injectable fillers

| Area | BNT-A | Fillers | Observation |
|---|---|---|---|
| Forehead lines | First | After if needed | BNT-A is usually enough |
| Glabella | First | After if needed | Fillers at this level are very beneficial for glabella reshaping. The duration of both procedures will be longer |
| Periorbital | First | After if needed | Fillers are barely needed at this area |
| Nasolabial fold | After if needed | First | The use of BNT-A should be done with caution to avoid asymmetries |
| Nose | To be used into the depressor septi nasi to block the drooping effect of muscle contraction | To be used into the nasal dorsum, at the fronto-nasal and nasolabial angle. | Their use may be concomitant with non-surgical reshape of the nose |
| Perioral | After if needed* | First | Usually fillers are enough in this area. The use of BNT-A is used to improve performance of result |
| Cheek | After if needed* | First | BNT-A injection in this area should be carried out with caution |
| Oral comissure | First if the main component results from muscle depression | First if the main component is tissue atrophy | The synergist use of both procedures is ideal in moderate to severe cases |
| Chin | First | After if chin enlargement is targeted | Skin wrinkling is more common than chin reshape with fillers |
| Neck | Ideal for platysma bands (vertical) | Ideal for moderate to deep horizontal lines | Both procedures can be undertaken in the same session |

* Some colleagues may start with BNT-A first if there is a strong muscular component

Cheek lines usually appear in advanced aging or earlier in patients with photo-damaged skin. The repeated contraction of the zygomaticus major and risorius on the thin or atrophic skin deepens the curvilinear cheek wrinkling. It is a typical facial area that presents both the static and dynamic component. In contrast to the glabella, for example, we do not want to block the muscle action completely, which would lead to functional impairment and atrophy. The use of fillers in such cases will lead to a thicker dermis. The single use of fillers, especially the biodegradable ones, may lead to quick absorption and diminish the result. The intradermal use of botulinum toxin on the cheek combined with fillers will enable the use of a smaller quantity of both products (see Sect. 6.3 on microinjections) (Fig. 8.3ab).

## 8.5  Botulinum Toxin and Brow Lift with Suspension Threads

The injection of botulinum toxin in the upper third before the use of suspension threads is quite new. As mentioned in the brow lift section (see Sect. 5.3), BNT-A may be used for lifting the brow, mainly its lateral parts. Surgical suspension threads (mersilene or prolene 3.0) are often used for lifting the brow, too. A blunt canulla of 2 mm is inserted at the m. frontalis level and the surgical thread is anchored into the subdermal or muscle layer below the brow hair. After the desired lifting effect is obtained, the thread is then sutured into the periosteum and/or the galea at the hairline level. An over-correction is usually undertaken.

The advantages of BNT-A treatment 2 weeks before placing the suspension threads includes the prior BNT-A-based lifting effect of the eyebrow and a better healing result through decreased movements due to paralysis of the m. frontalis and the depressors. But, above all, patients feel more confident about the effectiveness of both procedures (Fig. 8.4a,b).

## 8.6  Botulinum Toxin, Eye Surgery & Other Tiny Details

It is amazing to point out that the vast majority of patients still believe that the treatment of crow's feet is undertaken with blepharoplasty. The purpose of this cosmetic eye surgery is basically the removal of eye bags and skin excess. It is likely that with the resection of skin excess there will be a mild to moderate improvement in crow's feet wrinkling. However, we must make it clear to our patients that crow's feet result from muscle action and the proper treatment for this is BNT-A.

With medical development, we started to realize that there is not a single miraculous method that is able to correct all the complex alterations that may compromise the eye area. Surgery is beneficial for skin excess and eye bags, while BNT-A is useful for decreasing wrinkle formation. Some plastic surgeons inject BNT-A during surgery and report a longer-lasting result. There seems to be no harm for the surgical outcome if BNT-A is injected before surgery. However, some patients present unsatisfactory results if BNT-A is injected soon after the blepharoplasty during the edematous phase. It is advisable to inject BNT-A when edema subsides, which may mean 1–3 months after the surgery. Sometimes, patients are not aware that simple and tiny details make all the difference. The following pictures demonstrate what combined therapy may promote. (Fig. 8.5a,b)

## 8.7  Botulinum Toxin and Facelift

The advent of botulinum toxin has evidently changed the surgical approach to the face from the 1980s when very aggressive surgery with a coronal approach to the forehead was the rule, leading patients to complain about a very long downtime and sometimes an unnatural facial look.

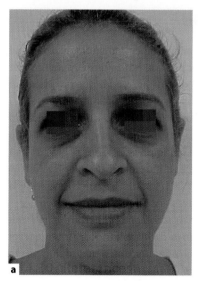
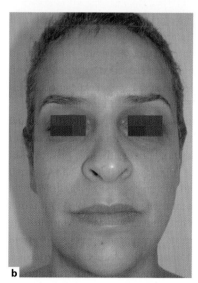

a    b

**Fig. 8.4a,b.** Patient with low lateral eyebrows and deep nasolabial folds. Before, and 15 days after, BNT-A in the upper third; fillers and BNT-A in the nasolabial fold and suspension surgical threads in the eyebrows. Note that the eyebrows remain over-corrected for the first 7 days. It is also important to tell the patient beforehand that BNT-A in the nasolabial fold may elongate the upper lip

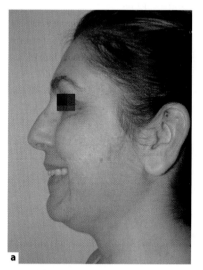
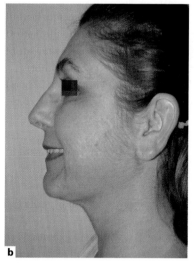

a    b

**Fig. 8.5a,b.** This patient presented a mild upper eyelid skin excess, a prominent nasal dorsum and fat deposit in the under chin. For treatment the patient's nose was reshaped using injectable fillers and BNT-A was injected into the m. depressor septi nasi. The neck was reshaped using chin liposuction. The upper third was treated with upper eyelid surgery followed by BNT-A injection into the crow's feet area

With the development of less and less invasive procedures, the upper third is now basically treated with BNT-A alone, which promotes rejuvenation improvement such as: brow lifting, erasing of horizontal lines in the forehead and vertical lines in the glabella area without scarring or downtime. So mini-lifts may focus basically on the middle and lower face and neck. Although mini-lifts are less invasive that the conventional facelift, a shorter but still not that short downtime is nevertheless an issue (Fig. 8.6a,b).

As the procedures are not undertaken at the same dermal level, all procedures may be done simultaneously.

## 8.8 The Microlift Procedure: BNT-A as an Important Ally!

The minimal approach technique (de Maio, 2004) was an innovation in facial cosmetic procedures that is faster, less painful, and less costly than surgical facelifts. The technique utilizes a variety of biodegradable injectable products and BNT-A to improve appearance with a fast and relatively painless lunchtime procedure. This lift has been expanded to the microlift procedure.

The microlift facelift appeals to the patient seeking a more long-lasting improvement than fillers and surface treatments offer but without the discomfort and cost of a surgical facelift. The technique utilizes three common treatments to improve facial contours: liposuction of the neck and under the chin, injection of facial fillers into wrinkles and folds, and suspension of facial muscles using polypropylene or mersilene threads. Alongside this, injection of botulinum toxin in the upper, mid and lower thirds is also a rule. Chemical peels can be added for some patients to further improve skin appearance. Patients appreciate that the microlift technique offers little scarring, minimal discomfort, and a quick recovery time. (Fig. 8.7a,b)

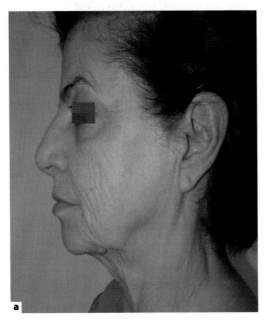
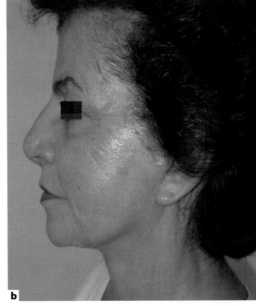

**Fig. 8.6a,b.** This patient presented intrinsic and extrinsic aging: saggy skin and excessive cheek wrinkling. After mini-lifting of the face and neck, a medium-depth chemical peel (TCA) and BNT-A in the upper third, a very natural and pleasant result was achieved

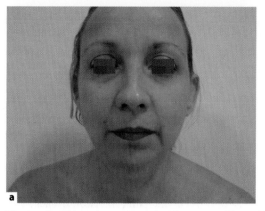 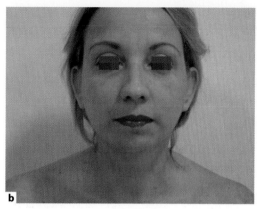

a    b

**Fig. 8.7a,b.** This patient presented with upper and lower blepharochalasis, deep nasolabial folds and oral comissures. In the mandible area, there is a mild presence of jowls. After microlifting, a blepharoplasty, BNT-A injections in the upper third, as well as injectable fillers for the eyebrows, nasolabial folds and oral commissures the patient presented a very natural result

Microlift Procedure
- BNT-A in the upper, mid and lower thirds
- Fillers for wrinkles, folds and nose re-shape fold
- Minimal skin undermining from a tiny incision in the inferior portion of the earlobe
- Surgical suspension threads (mersilene or prolene) for:
  - Jowls: always
  - Malar and eyebrow: if needed
- Liposuction of the chin
- Chemical peel or mild laser resurfacing: if needed

## 8.9  Tips and Tricks

■ Minimal invasive procedures are most important: put them all together! Be minimal and effective and give your patients a more complete treatment with a very short downtime.

## 8.10  References

Carruthers J et al. (2003) Deep resting glabellar rhytides respond to BTX-A and Hylan B. Dermatol Surg 29(5):539–44

Carruthers J, Carruthers A (2003) A prospective, randomized, parallel group study analyzing the effect of BTX-A (Botox) and nonanimal sourced hyaluronic acid (NASHA, Restylane) in combination compared with NASHA (Restylane) alone in severe glabellar rhytides in adult female subjects: treatment of severe glabellar rhytides with a hyaluronic acid derivative compared with the derivative and BTX-A. Dermatol Surg 29(8):802–9

Carruthers J, Carruthers A (2004) The effect of full-face broadband light treatments alone and in combination with bilateral crow's feet Botulinum toxin type A chemodenervation. Dermatol Surg 30(3):355–66; discussion p 366

Carruthers J, Carruthers A (2005) Facial sculpting and tissue augmentation. Dermatol Surg 31(11 Pt 2):1604–12

Coleman KR, Carruthers J (2006) Combination therapy with BOTOX trademark and fillers: the new rejuvenation paradigm. Dermatol Ther 19(3):177–88

de Maio M (2004) The minimal approach: an innovation in facial cosmetic procedures. Aesthetic Plast Surg 28(5):295–300. Epub 2004 Nov 4

Fagien S, Brandt FS (2001) Primary and adjunctive use of botulinum toxin type A (Botox) in facial aesthetic surgery: beyond the glabella. Clin Plast Surg 28(1):127–48

Fagien S (1999) Botox for the treatment of dynamic and hyperkinetic facial lines and furrows: adjunctive use in facial aesthetic surgery. Plast Reconstr Surg 103(2):701–13

Kikkawa DO, Kim JW (1997) Lower-eyelid blepharoplasty. Int Ophthalmol Clin 37(3):163–78

Guerrissi JO (2000) Intraoperative injection of botulinum toxin A into orbicularis oculi muscle for the treatment of crow's feet. Plast Reconstr Surg 105(6):2219–25; discussion pp 2226–8

Mole B (2003) Optimal forehead rejuvenation. Combining endoscopy-peel-botulinum toxin. Ann Chir Plast Esthet 48(3):143–51

Patel MP et al. (2004) Botox and collagen for glabellar furrows: advantages of combination therapy. Ann Plast Surg 52(5):442–7; discussion p 447

Semchyshyn NL, Kilmer SL (2005) Does laser inactivate botulinum toxin? Dermatol Surg 31(4):399–404

Yamauchi PS et al. (2004) Botulinum toxin type A gives adjunctive benefit to periorbital laser resurfacing. J Cosmet Laser Ther 6(3):145–8

Zimbler MS et al. (2001) Effect of botulinum toxin pretreatment on laser resurfacing results: a prospective, randomized, blinded trial. Arch Facial Plast Surg 3(3):165–9

Zimbler MS, Nassif PS (2003) Adjunctive applications for botulinum toxin in facial aesthetic surgery. Facial Plast Surg Clin North Am 11(4):477–82

8

# Subject Index

Printing: Krips bv, Meppel
Binding: Stürtz, Würzburg